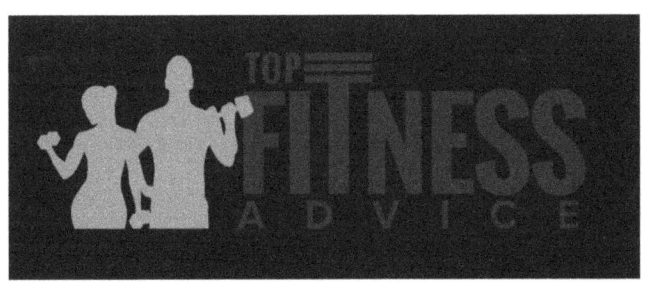

HEALTHY HABITS VOL. 2

17 EXTRA Morning Habits That Help You Lose Weight, Feel Energized & Live Healthy!

LINDA WESTWOOD

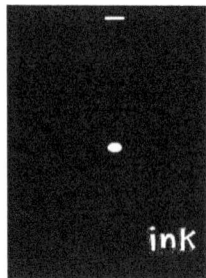

First published in 2015 by Venture Ink Publishing

Copyright © Top Fitness Advice 2019

All rights reserved.

No part of this book may be reproduced in any form without permission in writing from the author. No part of this publication may be reproduced or transmitted in any form or by any means, mechanic, electronic, photocopying, recording, by any storage or retrieval system, or transmitted by email without the permission in writing from the author and publisher.

Requests to the publisher for permission should be addressed to publishing@ventureink.co

For more information about the contents of this book or questions to the author, please contact Linda Westwood at linda@topfitnessadvice.com

Disclaimer

This book provides wellness management information in an informative and educational manner only, with information that is general in nature and that is not specific to you, the reader. The contents of this book are intended to assist you and other readers in your personal wellness efforts. Consult your physician regarding the applicability of any information provided in this book to you.

Nothing in this book should be construed as personal advice or diagnosis, and must not be used in this manner. The information provided about conditions is general in nature. This information does not cover all possible uses, actions, precautions, side-effects, or interactions of medicines, or medical procedures. The information in this book should not be considered as complete and does not cover all diseases, ailments, physical conditions, or their treatment.

You should consult with your physician before beginning any exercise, weight loss, or health care program. This book should not be used in place of a call or visit to a competent health-care professional. You should consult a health care professional before adopting any of the suggestions in this book or before drawing inferences from it.

Any decision regarding treatment and medication for your condition should be made with the advice and consultation of a qualified health care professional. If you have, or suspect you have, a health-care problem, then you should immediately contact a qualified health care professional for treatment.

No Warranties: The author and publisher don't guarantee or warrant the quality, accuracy, completeness, timeliness, appropriateness or suitability of the information in this book, or of any product or services referenced in this book.

The information in this book is provided on an "as is" basis and the author and publisher make no representations or warranties of any kind with respect to this information. This book may contain inaccuracies, typographical errors, or other errors.

Liability Disclaimer: The publisher, author, and other parties involved in the creation, production, provision of information, or delivery of this book specifically disclaim any responsibility, and shall not be held liable for any damages, claims, injuries, losses, liabilities, costs, or obligations including any direct, indirect, special, incidental, or consequences damages (collectively known as "Damages") whatsoever and howsoever caused, arising out of, or in connection with the use or misuse of the site and the information contained within it, whether such Damages arise in contract, tort, negligence, equity, statute law, or by way of other legal theory.

Table of Contents

Disclaimer	3
Who is this book for?	9
What will this book teach you?	11
Introduction	13
Important – Please read this before you begin…	15
EXTRA Morning Habit #1: Satiate Your Sweet Tooth	17
EXTRA Morning Habit #2: Keep THIS in Mind & Your Health Will Drastically Change	23
EXTRA Morning Habit #3: This ONE Thing Will Destroy ALL Progress You Could Make	29
EXTRA Morning Habit #4: The Most Annoying but IMPORTANT Morning Habit	31
EXTRA Morning Habit #5: Eat the RIGHT Fat	35
EXTRA Morning Habit #6: Add A Berry Booster	39
EXTRA Morning Habit #7: Add in Some of These Health-Boosters!	43
EXTRA Morning Habit #8: Start Your Breakfast with These Magic Ingredients	45
EXTRA Morning Habit #9: Release Tension	49

EXTRA Morning Habit #10: An EASY Habit with Exponential Benefits — 57

EXTRA Morning Habit #11: Have A Power Shower Every Morning — 61

EXTRA Morning Habit #12: Find A Fitness App That Suits YOU — 75

EXTRA Morning Habit #13: Mindful Eating — 79

EXTRA Morning Habit #14: Your Morning Pages — 83

EXTRA Morning Habit #15: The Simple Way to Achieve Zen — 89

EXTRA Morning Habit #16: Read Motivational Literature or Listen to It Daily — 93

EXTRA Morning Habit #17: Your Morning Meditation — 105

BONUS Morning Habit #18: Your Morning Visualization and Gratitude Session — 113

Final Words — 125

Would you prefer to listen to my book, rather than read it?

Download the audiobook version for free!

If you go to the special link below and sign up to Audible as a new customer, you can get the audiobook version of my book completely free.

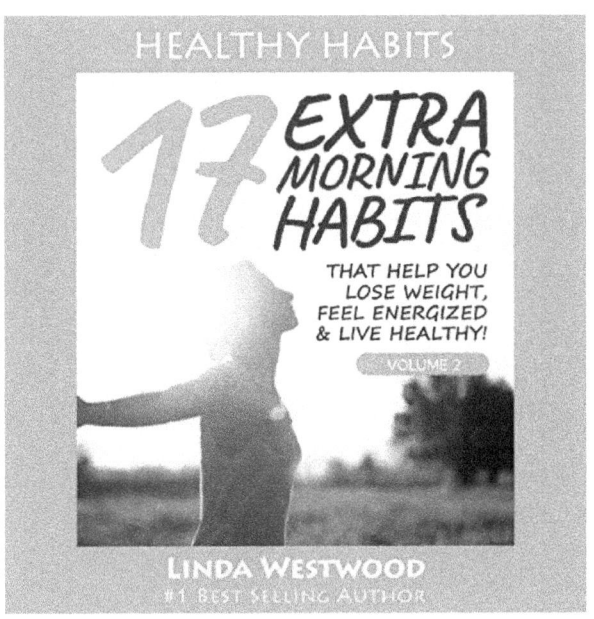

Go here to get your audiobook version for free:

TopFitnessAdvice.com/go/ExtraMorning

Who is this book for?

Have you tried to lose weight before but failed?

Are you struggling to stick to healthy habits?

Are you one of those people who *know* what to do, but struggle to *actually do* it?

Then this book is for you!

I am going to share with you some of the MOST effective morning habits that you can add into your life to lose weight, feel great and be energized throughout your entire day!

I have given you a simple action plan at the end of each chapter so you can implement each habit very easily!

Also, you don't have to be overweight to benefit from these habits.

Yes, they help you lose weight, but they also help you live a healthy life, as well as feel recharged and energized ALL DAY LONG!

What will this book teach you?

This book is not like others!

It doesn't just contain generic advice that we all already know, but actual morning habits that have been identified to INCREASE weight loss, IMPROVE energy levels, and LEAD to a more healthy life!

Some of these habits are very simple and you can begin implementing them from tomorrow morning, and some are a little more difficult, in that you will need to practice them more!

I will also share with you why each of these habits work and are so effective – along with a simple action plan to help get you started and on your way to lasting success!

Introduction

Want to lose weight and feel great?

Then this is the book for you.

If you are anything like me, you have tried just about every diet on the planet and have lost and regained weight several times over.

It's a vicious cycle – you diet and lose the fat, only to find that it arrives back with MORE when the diet is over!

Diets don't work!

They create an unnatural feeling of deprivation and the body starts to rebel quite fast.

I, for example, am not a choc-a-holic – I enjoy chocolates, but don't eat too many of them... until I go on a diet.

Once I start a diet my body starts demanding chocolates, and all the other stuff I shouldn't be eating.

Many people find that the same type of thing happens to them. Dieting is clearly not the answer. If dieting did work, there would only be one diet plan out there and no one would be overweight or obese.

This book is different – it is not a diet book.

In this book I give you 17 little habits that you can add into your lifestyle so that you naturally and painlessly lose weight and keep it off.

Seventeen may seem like a lot but here's the rub – you will adopt each one individually, at your own pace. In fact, I insist that you do not rush it – this process should take no less than two weeks at the very least.

I know that you are motivated to get started on everything now, but this program works because it is done step-by-step. Introducing each habit individually allows your body to cope more readily with the changes. Try to do them all at once and you will probably give up.

Each habit will, by itself, help you to lose weight. As you build more habits in, each habit builds on the last and you will see even more progress.

Some habits will be easier to adopt than others but, at the end of the day, it is worthwhile to adopt all of them.

Eventually, when you have adopted all the habits, you will be living at the next level – you'll be healthier and more energetic in ways that you have never been before.

Read the book slowly, I have written out an action plan for each habit to make it easy for you.

No more excuses – let's dive right in!

Important – Please read this before you begin…

This book is an extension to the original **Healthy Habits: The 13 Morning Habits That Can Help You to Lose Weight, Feel More Energized & Live A Healthier Life!**

13 Morning Habits was a MASSIVE hit worldwide that became a #1 best seller in over 9 different book categories (all under Health & Fitness).

Since then, I have gone ahead and written health & fitness books on many other topics, but nothing has been as successful as the original **13 Morning Habits** – in fact, all my fans have constantly asked for an extended edition.

Finally, I gave in!

And the result is this fantastic, well put-together book that you are about to read. I would like to officially thank all my fans that have continued to read my books and follow me.

IMPORTANT: If you haven't already read the original, **Healthy Habits: The 13 Morning Habits That Can Help You to Lose Weight, Feel More Energized & Live A Healthier Life!**, I strongly recommend reading it before you read this, because this book acts as a 2nd volume in the series.

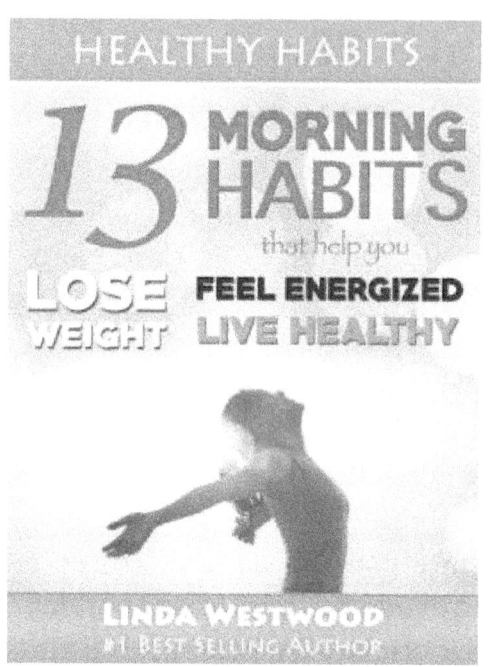

Check Out "13 Morning Habits"!

EXTRA Morning Habit #1

Satiate Your Sweet Tooth

One of the worst things about being on a diet is that you have a whole range of restrictions on what you can and cannot eat. If, like me, you have a bit of a sweet tooth, this can be very problematic.

The good news is that you do not have to give up on sweetness altogether, as long as you moderate your intake.

Dark chocolate is a great way to get a taste of the "good" life, boost your antioxidant levels and also help to keep you healthy. Dark chocolate, with at least 70% cocoa solids is a source of healthy monounsaturated fats and these, in turn, can help your body to improve the amount of belly fat used.

Belly fat is particularly unhealthy as the fat is concentrated around the organs. It has been linked to an increased risk of the development of lifestyle diseases such as heart disease and diabetes and can be difficult to shift.

So, I am saying that you can eat dark chocolate with your breakfast – the catch? That you can only eat 4 squares of it and that it has to have at least 70% cocoa solids, more if possible. You must also either have it with breakfast or after breakfast but never on an empty stomach. Eating it on an empty stomach will push your blood sugar levels up too high, negating the benefits of having monounsaturated fats.

Personally, I love the taste of chocolate in the morning – I will quite often eat breakfast for supper and supper at breakfast time – but not everyone is like that.

If the idea of having chocolate so early in the morning is one that does not sit well with you, find fun ways to incorporate it. Grate it into your oatmeal or melt it and use it as a dip for strawberries. Just incorporate it.

Get Some Honey, Honey

Oh, bother – Winnie the Pooh was right all along – honey is yummy and can be very good for you. Where silly old Pooh does get it wrong though is that he eats too much of it and he eats it on its own.

If chocolate simply will not work for you in the morning but you still have a sweet tooth, adding a little honey to sweeten things up for you can work as well.

Again, remember that honey is basically just pure sugar and so it will cause spikes in your blood sugar if eaten on its own. The advantage that honey has over sugar is that it is a lot more nutritious and can help the body to heal. (Honey is the only cough medicine that we use in our house.)

Mix it in with your green tea to give it a flavor boost or mix it in with your porridge, muesli, etc.

Raw honey is the better option as it has not been irradiated and contains more nutrients. Do be careful when selecting the brand that you will use. You want honey that has not been diluted to make it go further.

A Cautionary Tale

There is one caveat when it comes to including honey or chocolate in your diet in this manner – if this leads to craving more sugar, or if you cannot pull yourself back from eating just a little bit of the chocolate a day, you need to cut it out completely.

Sometimes the call of sugar can be too strong and, if this is the case for you, it is better to start cutting it out of your life completely. We will deal with more about doing this in the next chapter.

ACTION PLAN

1. Get yourself a slab or two of dark chocolate.

2. Break it up into portions of 4 pieces each.

3. Keep only two portions at a time in the refrigerator and freeze the rest. (This will help you to prevent binge eating as the chocolate needs to be defrosted before eating it.)

4. If you want to, you can grate the chocolate over your morning oats in order to sweeten them.

5. Alternatively, look for some raw honey.

Discover Scientifically-Proven "Shortcuts" & "Hacks" to Lose Weight FASTER (With Very Little Effort)

For this month only, you can get Linda's best-selling & most popular book absolutely free – *Weight Loss Secrets You NEED to Know.*

Get Your FREE Copy Here:
TopFitnessAdvice.com/Bonus

Discover scientifically-proven tips to help you lose weight faster and easier than ever before. With this book, readers were able to improve their weight loss results and fitness levels. So, it's highly recommended that you get this book, especially while it's free!

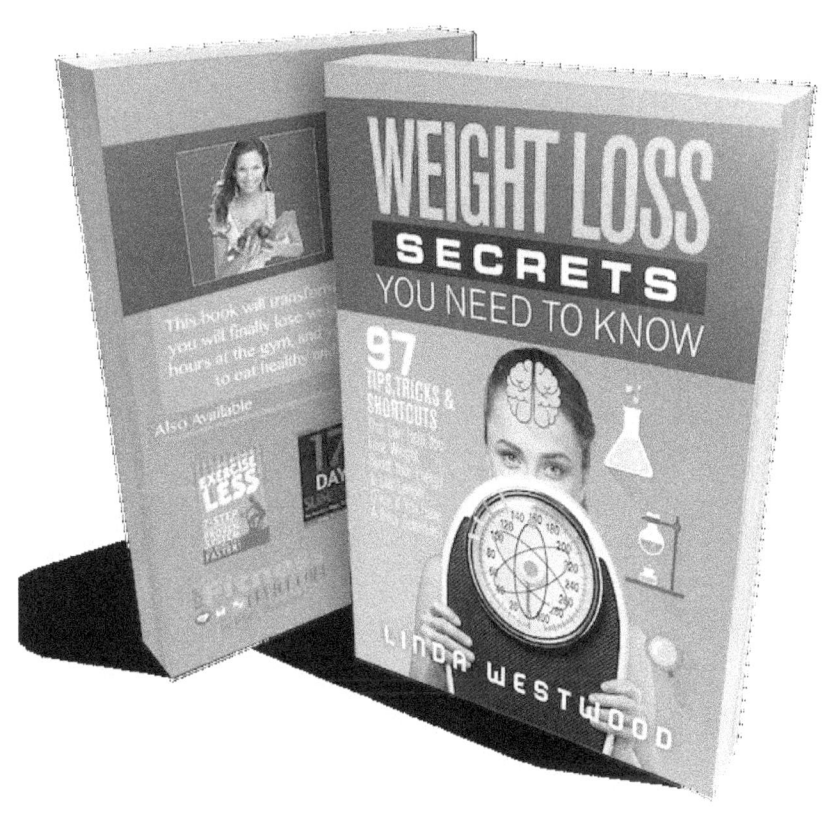

Get Your FREE Copy Here:
TopFitnessAdvice.com/Bonus

EXTRA Morning Habit #2

Keep THIS in Mind & Your Health Will Drastically Change

By now you are probably aware that refined sugar is really bad for you. Did you know, however, that the average American has around 22 teaspoons of sugar a day?

Think that I am exaggerating? Open your grocery cupboard and have a look at the list of ingredients. Most tinned foods – even things like soup – will have some form of sugar in them. Not even bacon escapes – it is often cured using syrup or sugar.

Refined sugar is one of the most dangerous foodstuffs (and I use that term loosely) on the planet. It is added to most processed foods in order to improve the taste and the main problem is that it plays havoc with your blood sugar levels.

Another cause for concern is that sugar acts on the same pleasure centers in the brain that narcotics do and so you can become addicted to it just as easily.

This, combined with the impact of it on your blood sugar means that you not only get hungry faster after eating it but that you actually can become addicted to it as well.

As a result, it is far better for your health to cut it out completely.

Now, this may seem like contradictory advice considering that I just told you that you can eat dark chocolate but it really is not. Dark chocolate contains less added sugar than other forms of chocolate and you are consuming only a few squares a day, after a big meal so the impact on your blood sugar levels is minimal.

If having dark chocolate in the morning helps to prevent you craving sweets and feeling deprived later on in the day, the benefits far outweigh any potential risks.

The same cannot be said for sugar added to coffee, or breakfast cereals that are packed with sugar. (And believe me, a lot of the so-called healthy cereals are packed with sugar – even the bran flakes – because sugar makes them taste better.) You would be better off eating cardboard than some of the sugar-laden cereals on the market.

By avoiding too much sugar in the morning, you are reducing the chances of your blood sugar levels crashing later in the day and so are more likely to be able to stick to your healthy eating plan.

Try this experiment today, just do not add any sugar into your coffee or tea and make sure not to add it in anywhere else. Now go cold turkey for a couple of days – how did you end up feeling? Chances are good that you started out feeling as though you needed a sugar rush. Perhaps you had less energy than normal. This is a normal reaction to cutting back on your sugar intake as a whole and is basically caused by your body going into withdrawal.

If you want to cut your sugar intake completely, or want to restrict it only to the pieces of chocolate, you can choose to either go cold turkey or cut sugar out over a longer period.

The approach you choose will depend on what works best for you and how much sugar you have been consuming already.

If you have been having two sodas a day, three sugars in your coffee and sugary cereal for breakfast, it is going to be harder to kick the habit, especially if you just cut it out completely.

And that is where these morning habits can really help you out – remember how, at the beginning of this book, I advised you to adopt the habits slowly so that there was not as much of a shock to the system? The same applies to cutting back on sugar.

The cold turkey approach will work for some but not for others – the problem I have with the cold turkey approach is that you end up feeling quite horrible for about a week or so and it can be tough to keep up your motivation to stop eating added sugar. It can also be a huge adjustment to go from having two or three spoons of sugar in your coffee to none overnight.

The good news is that you can retrain your taste-buds over time so that you gradually become accustomed to eating foods that are not as sweet.

Kicking the Sugar Habit

If you opt for reducing your sugar intake slowly, reduce it over a three-week period for optimal results. This allows you to wean yourself off sugar more slowly and helps you to avoid that nasty backlash of withdrawal symptoms. It is important to watch out for sugar in all its forms. You would be surprised exactly how many foods do contain sugar. If a food is processed, there is a high probability that it does have added sugar. Commercial peanut butters, for example, usually have sugar in them as well.

Week 1: Halve the amount of soda that you drink and reduce the amount of sugar in your coffee/ tea by half as well. This is the week for reducing the amount of sugar you take in in the form of beverages. Get rid of sugar to be used in coffee/ tea, sodas and check your creamer as well – it is likely to have sugar in it.

Week 2: Cut out the sugary snacks and desserts. If you are really battling to cope without the sugar, add in some fresh fruit snacks. One word here – whilst dried fruit is a better option than candy, it is only a slightly better option. Dried fruit does have some vitamins, minerals and fiber but also has a lot of sugar in it. The sugar in the dried fruits negates any benefits of the nutrients and fiber. You are better off eating the whole fruit – the sugars are a lot less concentrated and the water content will help you to feel full for a lot longer as well.

Week 3: Toss out processed foods and any other foods that contain high levels of added sugar. Check through your cupboards and make sure that all sugar is gone. The only sugar that you should have left in your house is in the form of natural fruits and your dark chocolate, if you are continuing with that.

The great news is that, while it may be hard to kick a sugar addiction at first, once you are over it, it becomes a lot easier to live without it. You will feel more energized, healthier and look better all for simply kicking added sugar out of your life.

You will start to see the benefits in as little as two weeks and, once you are off sugar for good, you will not really even want to go back.

Considering the negative effect that added sugar has on the metabolism, the fact that it is full of empty calories and the fact that it can actually contribute to the toxic load within the body, ditching sugar is one of the best health moves that you can make for yourself and your family as a whole.

ACTION PLAN

1. Check your cereal to see what the sugar content is.

2. Stop buying refined sugar – if you don't have any, you cannot use it.

3. Get rid of sugary cereals and sugar that you have in your cupboard.

4. Go cold turkey when it comes to your morning tea or coffee – the dark chocolate will be enough to help you satiate your sweet tooth in the interim.

EXTRA Morning Habit #3

This ONE Thing Will Destroy ALL Progress You Could Make

Recent research has shown that some artificial sweeteners, such as aspartame, can be carcinogenic and that those that are not actually do more harm than good anyway – the body is not fooled by these sweeteners at all and will still crave sugar, despite the fact that you are ingesting them. You are better off cutting artificial sweeteners out of your diet altogether.

Add in the potential digestive upsets that can be caused by ingesting too much of these sweeteners and they become an even less attractive option.

Some natural sweeteners are little better than refined sugar in terms of their effects on your blood sugar level. Agave syrup, for example, is completely natural but full of carbs and so can play havoc with your sugar levels.

If you absolutely have to use a sweetener of some type or another, Stevia is your best bet. Stevia is an herb and sweeteners derived from it are sweeter than sugar. If you have a problem with unstable blood sugar levels, this could be the solution for you as Stevia not only sweetens your food and beverages but also plays an active role in helping the body to regulate insulin production.

Stevia is available in extract form quite widely but it can also pay to plant it in your garden. It is a relatively easy plant to grow and, once established, very undemanding. Simply pick a leaf or two as necessary to sweeten your morning cup of green tea to get the benefits. Alternatively, use the extract.

ACTION PLAN

1. Remove all artificial sweeteners from your grocery cupboard and get rid of them.

2. If you do require a sweetener of some sort, look for a Stevia-based one.

3. Check all products that you buy to ensure that they have not been artificially sweetened. Many low-fat yoghurts, etc. have been artificially sweetened.

I hope that you are enjoying this book so far, and if you could spare 30 seconds, I would greatly appreciate you leaving a review on Amazon.com.

EXTRA Morning Habit #4

The Most Annoying but IMPORTANT Morning Habit

Good dental hygiene is one of those habits that we know we need to follow through with but one that many people do end up rushing or skipping, especially if rushed for time. Most people understand the dangers of tooth decay – that left unchecked you could develop gingivitis or periodontal disease and end up losing your teeth. What less people are aware of is the link between the bacteria on the teeth and cardiovascular disease.

Brushing your teeth soon after your morning breakfast is a healthy habit that can help to protect you against not only tooth decay but also against heart disease. A build-up of plaque on the teeth has been linked to an increased risk of heart disease and inflammation in the body.

Plaque is basically a bacteria, and if allowed to grow unchecked, this bacteria can cross into the blood stream leading to inflammation and plaque formation in the blood vessels. This, in turn, can lead to cardiovascular problems like heart disease and strokes.

You need to starve the plaque of food as much as possible and this means clearing out any remnants of food after a meal. Rinsing out your mouth after a meal will help but is not enough.

In order to clear off the plaque, you need to brush your teeth for at least two minutes, being sure to do a thorough job and to get a full mouth clean. It is important to clean your teeth thoroughly without actually pressing too hard on the gums – applying a soft pressure with the toothbrush at a 45-degree angle to the teeth is the most effective angle to use.

Flossing between each of the teeth is another important aspect of gum health. The toothbrush simply cannot reach all the small spaces between your teeth and so you need to floss to ensure that as much debris as possible is cleaned out. You need to wind a piece of floss around two fingers and then gently push it into the space between your teeth in order to get out any leftover debris.

I also follow up flossing with a quick brushing of the teeth again – this time not using any toothpaste, just a damp toothbrush. This removes any specks of debris loosened by flossing and is important for a complete mouth cleansing.

Follow this up with brushing or scraping your tongue. You can, if you like, buy a special tongue scraper but I have been using my toothbrush to clean my tongue for years and I find that a scraper would be extraneous and just add more clutter to the bathroom.

Follow up with a good rinse and you are ready to go. You can choose to use a mouthwash or not, as you prefer. After a few weeks of proper brushing though, a mouthwash will generally be unnecessary. If you do decide to continue to use one, be sure to choose one that does not have alcohol in it at all.

Alcohol in the mix does help to kill off bacteria in the mouth but it is also very drying and can thus undermine gum health. It is not necessary to use an alcohol-based mouthwash as long as you are cleaning your teeth effectively every day.

ACTION PLAN

1. Check your toothbrush for signs of wear – if you are brushing your teeth as you should, your toothbrush should last between 3 and 6 months.

2. Make sure that you have a supply of dental floss. If you find it difficult to figure out how to maneuver the floss, look for a dental floss dispenser or pre-loaded floss picks that make it a lot easier to floss.

3. You can buy a tongue scraper if you like but I simply use my toothbrush to clean my tongue.

EXTRA Morning Habit #5

Eat the RIGHT Fat

Research is now showing that the low-fat craze that has been advocated as the healthiest way to eat over the last few decades is actually not an effective way to lose weight at all. The average person is now heavier than was the case 50 years ago and obesity has become a growing global epidemic.

More than that, the low-fat diets seem to have done more harm than good. The problem with foods that have had the fat removed is that they simply do not taste as good. To help counter the loss of flavor, these foods usually have a lot of added sugar.

And the added sugar is a lot more dangerous for you than a bit of extra fat. Fat is a lot more satisfying to eat whereas sugar only leaves you craving the next sugar rush.

We have, as a society, dropped the levels of fat in our diet but replaced it with a far more dangerous element – sugar.

And it is not only the sugar that becomes a problem – most of these foods are also highly processed and loaded with synthetic chemicals.

The combination is deadly – the added sugar plays havoc with your blood sugar levels, eventually causing your body to become less sensitive to insulin. The chemicals increase the toxic load on your system, making it harder for your body to keep up.

That is only the tip of the iceberg though. Research has now also shown that those who eat full fat dairy in place of low fat dairy are less likely to be obese. Scientists believe that the reason for this is that the fatty acids that are removed to make the dairy low fat play a role in appetite and hormone regulation.

Scientists also believe that this again boils down to whole food versus processed food – the micronutrients within the whole dairy working well together. Mother Nature is one of the best scientists in the world – she knows what will work and what will not. Whole foods have the ideal balance of nutrients and by removing some of those elements, we are making the food less nutritious overall.

The upshot? Eat full fat dairy with your breakfast – research has shown that this will help to keep you feeling fuller for longer and will help to influence the way that your body burns calories.

As far as possible, try to source dairy products from pasture fed and organically raised cattle as these foods are healthier and more nutritious than the others.

Look for milk, yoghurt, cream and butter to eat with your breakfast and make sure that there are no artificial sweeteners or any added sugars. It is easy to begin to incorporate more full-fat dairy. Simply add a glass of milk in as part of your meal or mix in some yoghurt with your oatmeal.

If you are frying your breakfast, use butter as your cooking oil. Everything tastes better with a bit of butter in it. You can also start to add cream back into your daily routine. I make omelets some days for breakfast and use a little cream in the egg mixture in place of milk. I then fry the omelet in pure butter.

It is important to get non-flavored yoghurt as the other kind can be packed with sugar – a small tub of yoghurt can contain as much sugar as a soda does and so it is really not the healthier option at all.

If you cannot bear the thought of eating plain yoghurt, you can improve the flavor using a little bit of honey – no more than a half a teaspoon per 175ml tub, mind you. Alternatively mix in chopped up fresh fruit and nuts to boost the flavor of the yoghurt.

The overall benefit of eating full fat dairy again is that you will not only feel fuller but the food will also taste so much better as well. This can come in very handy when you are practicing mindful eating. (I will tell you more about mindful eating further down the page.)

ACTION PLAN

1. Look for a source of organic, pasture-fed dairy products. Try your local farmer's market.

2. Finish or get rid of any low-fat dairy products and replace with full fat alternatives.

3. Replace margarine and low-fat spreads with real butter.

EXTRA Morning Habit #6

Add A Berry Booster

For another big boost of antioxidants, without adding a whole lot of unnecessary carbs, add in a half a cup of the berries of your choice. If possible, grow your own berries – I grow my own strawberries and raspberries and they taste a whole lot better than those that you can get commercially.

If growing your own is not an option, try to find a local farmer, preferably one that employs organic farming methods and order the berries in bulk – I do this because we eat more berries than what we can produce overall. Buying in bulk is a little bit of work initially – you need to repack and freeze the berries yourself but it usually works out a lot less expensive overall and you have more control over how fresh the berries are.

If neither of the above are an option, or berries are out of season, get yourself some frozen berries so that you always have them on hand. Frozen berries can be mixed in with oatmeal or blended into a smoothie for a real anti-oxidant boost.

It is also important to switch out the type of berries that you eat from time to time so that you can vary the nutrients contained in your food overall. That means that if you eat blueberries today, try to eat raspberries tomorrow and strawberries the next day, etc.

Berries can also help to regulate blood sugar levels – they are typically lower in sugars and have a high fiber count making them one of the healthiest fruits that you can consume.

The tarter the berries are, the less natural sugar they contain. That said, even sweet berries are lower in natural sugar and so can be enjoyed.

If you want a warmer breakfast option, consider making a berry coulis to add to your porridge. All that a berry coulis essentially is is the berries simmered in a bit of water until they become soft and more like jelly. Traditionally one would add sugar as well but this step can be left out with little trouble.

Once the coulis has cooled, you can also mix it into your yoghurt for added flavor or you could freeze it to add to smoothies at a later stage.

I love a berry smoothie in summer and they are so easy to make.

Ingredients

- 1 tub of berries of your choice, hulled and well rinsed
- 1 medium banana, peeled, frozen
- 1 carrot scrubbed and chopped – you won't even taste it
- A handful of almonds
- A cup of milk or water

Method

1. Blend everything together for a wonderful berry smoothie and drink and enjoy.

ACTION PLAN

1. If you have space in your garden, consider planting some berries – when they start to produce, be sure to protect them against birds – they also love the taste of fresh berries.

2. If you cannot grow enough, look at your local farmer's market in season to supplement your supply.

3. Alternatively, source frozen berries and keep them in your freezer, ready for when you need them.

Once again, thank you for reading this book, and I hope you're getting a lot of valuable information. I would greatly appreciate it if you could take 30 seconds to leave me a review for this book on Amazon.com.

EXTRA Morning Habit #7

Add in Some of These Health-Boosters!

All of us have bacteria that grow in our intestinal tracts – some beneficial, others less so. In a healthy person, these bacteria balance each other out and we have a healthy digestive system.

This balance is fairly easy to upset though and, when this happens, the beneficial bacteria can soon become outnumbered. The problem with this is that you then have less protection in terms of what passes through the gut and into the bloodstream. Basically, what happens is that harmful substances from our food that, when you are healthy, would be retained in the gut until expelled leak over into the bloodstream causing inflammation and allergic reactions.

When the gut bacteria are not balanced, you can expect to see an increase in inflammatory conditions, such as rheumatism, etc. and expect to feel bloated and a lot less energetic. Your immune system will also become compromised.

The best way to overcome these conditions is to carefully monitor which foods cause problems and which create them. Sugar is, again, a villain here and can stimulate the growth of harmful bacteria, throwing the gut system out of whack again.

Fortunately, restoring the balance is not that hard as the cells in the gut take less than a week to completely replace themselves. By adopting better eating habits now, you can turn this situation around and ensure that you have a healthier digestive system and, if you have already started adopting the habits laid out in this book, you will already be on your way.

Kick recovery up a notch by including yoghurt with the following healthy bacteria in it – acidophilus and bifidus. Unsweetened Greek yoghurt is best and, if you can, get yoghurt made from the milk of pasture-fed cattle.

Alternatively, you can take a pro-biotic supplement for a short while as well.

It is also a good idea to take in extra pro-biotics if you are ill or if you need to take antibiotics. Just be sure not to take the antibiotics at the same time as your pre-biotics.

To maintain a healthy gut, you need to ensure that you get the right amount of fiber, cut back on sugar intake and get a variety of fresh foods, eaten as close to their natural state as possible.

ACTION PLAN

1. Look for natural Greek yoghurt, unsweetened at your local store. Organic is best.

2. If you have not done so already, start increasing your fiber intake.

3. End each breakfast off with a small tub of yoghurt.

EXTRA Morning Habit #8

Start Your Breakfast with These Magic Ingredients

When it comes to promoting healthy digestion, there is little better that you can do than to eat raw food as far as possible. Raw food contains some digestive enzymes that can help promote good digestion.

These enzymes, however, can be destroyed by cooking so, where you can, it is best to eat raw foods. In addition, cooking will also break down some of the fiber in the food and this, again, is not good for promoting a healthy digestive system.

Raw food can help to feed the healthy bacteria in the gut and so restore balance.

Prebiotics can help to feed the healthy bacteria in the gut without overdosing your system. Prebiotics are basically foods that are high in fiber and more difficult for the body to digest. Because of this, these substances pass through the stomach and are processed in the gut.

Prebiotics that can be of use include lentils, beans and chickpeas.

Chickpeas can be enjoyed in a number of different ways and are a very versatile snack food. Roast some chickpeas in the oven with a drizzle of olive oil and seasoning to taste for a healthy alternative to crisps. Alternatively, you can cook the chickpeas and incorporate them into you morning smoothie or make them into hummus.

It is better to buy raw chickpeas and to cook them yourself as then you avoid the preservatives and salt present in the canned varieties. Just do be sure to soak them overnight and remove any that float or you could have a problem with gas.

The easiest way to incorporate these foods into your diet when raw is to grow your own sprouts. Sprouts are easy and quick to grow – all you need is a bottle and some muslin to cover the opening of the jar.

Cover the seeds in water and soak for about half an hour. Strain off the water and leave the sprouts in a cool, dark place. Repeat every morning and evening until the seeds start to sprout – depending on the seed this can be in as little as 3 -5 days. Mung beans and alfalfa will grow in two or three days, chickpeas can take a week.

Whilst not strictly necessary, I did find that a seed sprouter was a good investment to make and I do advise you to consider getting one yourself if you find that you enjoy sprouting vegetables.

The sprouter has a series of trays that are perforated to make it easy for water to drain off the sprouts. You simply place your sprouts on the trays and pour water over the top layer. The water filters down through all the layers and the excess collects in the tray for this purpose. The trays make things more convenient because they nestle on top of one another neatly and they allow you to more easily separate out your different sprouts. I have five trays going at any one time to ensure a steady supply of sprouts and enough variety.

When the seeds have grown about a centimeter, they are ready to eat. Eat at least a handful at a time – they provide amazing amounts of energy and are amongst the most nutritious foods on the planet. The leftovers can stay in the bottle or tray and will grow as long as you keep watering them. For best benefits though, eat within a couple of days of sprouting.

It is important to use food quality seeds for sprouting and not seeds intended for planting. Seeds that are intended for planting have usually been treated with poisons to help them stay healthy.

ACTION PLAN

1. Find a source of mung beans and raw chickpeas. We get great quality seeds at our local spice shop but you can also usually find them at your health shop.

2. Start off sprouting seeds in a bottle – if you like the flavor of the sprouts, get yourself a sprouter.

3. Look for alternative cooking methods – the more raw food that you can eat, the more pre-biotics you will take in overall.

EXTRA Morning Habit #9

Release Tension

This works best when done as a cool-down exercise after your cardio session. It is a combination of muscle stretching, muscle tension and muscle relaxation. It will help to remove any tension left over in the body after your exercise.

The whole exercise takes about 15-20 minutes overall. If you have back problems, do consult your health care practitioner before attempting these exercises.

Start by standing up straight, feet about a little apart and arms at your sides. Keep the whole body loose and limber and make sure that knees are not locked into place.

Imagine that a string is holding you up from the ceiling pulling your body with it – stretch your arms up over your head and stretch as high as you can, trying to reach the top-point of this "string".

Hold the stretch and carry on deepening it by standing on tip toes as well. (This may be tough at first but do persevere and you will get it right.) Hold the stretch for a few seconds and then return to your starting position. Repeat twice.

Now it is time to loosen up the neck. Look to your left, moving only your head. Hold for a few seconds. Roll the head in a smooth, even motion, keeping your chin as close to your chest as possible, until you are looking to your right. Repeat the exercise, this time reversing the action. This will help release tension in the neck.

Next bed from the waist and attempt to touch your toes. If you cannot, you can bend your knees slightly to assist. If you still cannot touch your toes at this point, you can just stop this exercise here and repeat daily until you can touch your toes.

Walk your fingers, still touching the floor, as far ahead of your toes as you can comfortably stretch. This should be a gentle stretch. Now walk your fingers backwards through your legs, as far back as you can comfortably manage. Walk your fingers back to the point just ahead of your toes. This helps to give the vertebrae an even deeper stretch.

Bend your knees so that you are on all fours. Pull in your belly. Arch your back as high as you comfortably can and hold for a count of 3. Come back to the starting position. Now curve your back so that your belly is lowered. Hold for a count of three and go back to starting position. Repeat the whole exercise a total of 3 times. This will help to release any tension help in the back.

Now kneel, with your back straight and buttocks on your lower legs. Extend your arms up as high as they will go, extending the stretch to ensure that your buttocks are also lifted off the ground. While at the top of the stretch, arch your back and moving your extended arms backwards to really get more of a stretch in. Return to the starting position. This helps to relieve tension held in the shoulders.

Now swap positions – you want to sit on the floor, back straight and legs extended out in front of you. With your right hand, grasp the outer edge of your left knee and, using this as a support, swivel your whole upper body around to the left. Hold for a few seconds before returning to the start. Repeat on the opposite side.

Do this exercise a total of 4 times. This is actually a yoga move and it has a number of benefits, for starters the spine is stretched and tension is released and, secondly the internal organs are lightly massaged, aiding with toning them and helping to move waste out of the body.

Return to the starting position and now concentrate on your feet. Using just the ankle, rotate the feet first clockwise and then counterclockwise five times each. Stretch out your toes and point as hard as you can with your feet. Hold for a couple of seconds and then release. Now flex your feet so that you can feel the action in your calf muscles. Hold for a few seconds and release. Do these pointing and flexing exercises five times each.

Now lie flat on the floor, with your knees bent. Slowly open your knees out towards the floor on either side of your body, feeling the stretch in the inner thighs. Carry on until the stretch is quite intense but not extremely uncomfortable. Bring your knees back together again and repeat 5 times.

Bring both knees up to the chest and hug them so that you feel the stretch in your hamstrings. Release and repeat 5 times.

Now lie flat on the ground for a few minutes, just breathing in and out deeply and then you are done.

Deep Relaxation

Now this is an exercise that you can do in the morning if you have a bit more time to spend and it is a particularly good one if you have had a restless night or bad night's sleep. Be warned, it is extremely relaxing so if you feel sleepy, set the alarm so that you wake up again if you nod off.

Whilst I would not do this every morning, this is a great exercise for you to do when you feel that you need to relax and recharge a bit.

Dress comfortably in non-constricting clothes and lie down flat. The floor is the ideal place for this exercise as the bed may be too comfortable. You need to place your arms loosely at your sides and position your legs a little apart from one another.

Take a few seconds to feel the sensation of your body touching the floor and sensing where you are carrying tension in your body.

Close your eyes and breathe in deeply through your nose. While you are breathing in, concentrate on your feet. As you breathe out, wriggle your feet a bit, making sure alternate flexing and pointing. Relax your feet and, as you do so, feel the tension flowing out of them into the floor. Your feet will start to feel heavier and lot more relaxed.

Repeat this exercise with your calves, then your thighs and then your hips, all the while imagining the tension and any pain present flowing out of your limbs and into the floor with every exhalation.

Move up to the belly and take a few deep breaths, again imagining the tension flowing out of your belly and into the floor.

Repeat with the chest and neck before moving onto the shoulders, arms and hands. Throughout this whole process, the areas that are relaxed should start to feel very heavy.

Finish off by concentrating on doing the same for your head. If you can, imagine the tension dripping off your scalp as well.

End off by checking each area again for any left-over tension, repeating the exercise as necessary in those areas where there is still some tension.
Now concentrate on the feeling of complete relaxation as you imagine your whole body becoming heavy and relaxed. Lay in that pose for about 5 minutes, concentrating of the feelings of relaxation.

If you start to feel bored, it is time to call it quits. Bring yourself out of it by moving your hands and feet again and stretching your limbs thoroughly.

Once that is done you can open your eyes and sit up slowly. Stretch again thoroughly before standing and, once you are up, stretch one last time.

ACTION PLAN

1. Look for either a yoga mat or a beach towel to use when doing these stretching exercises.

2. If you have issues with your back, and would like to try these exercises anyway, take this book along to your doctor's office and ask for their opinion.

3. Start out small with these exercises and gradually increase the stretch until your body becomes more limber overall.

Others who are considering purchasing this book would love to know what you think. If you could spare a few seconds, they would greatly appreciate reading an honest review from you. Simply visit the page on Amazon.com.

Enjoying this book?

Check out my other best sellers!

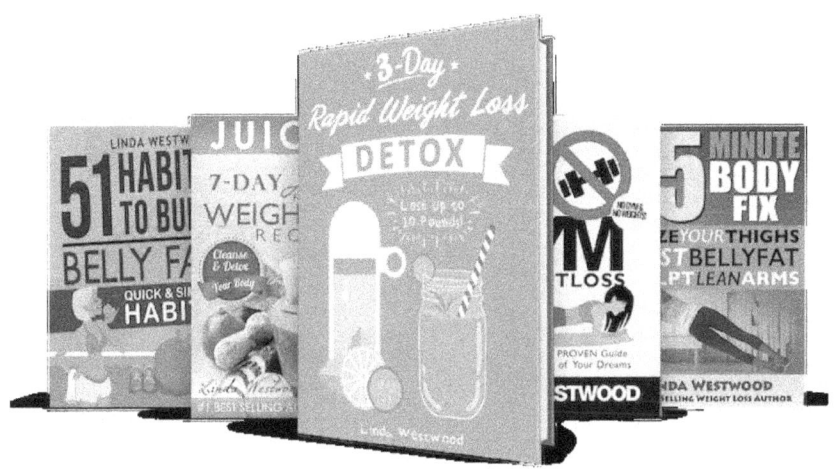

Get your next book on sale here:

TopFitnessAdvice.com/go/books

EXTRA Morning Habit #10

An EASY Habit with Exponential Benefits

This next habit may seem a bit of a funny one, considering that you have already been doing some form of cardio and stretching but the goal here is not to get exercise, although you will, but more to get you out and about into nature and into the sunlight.

You will walk out without any sunscreen on and let the sun's rays kiss your skin. Many people today are deficient in Vitamin D – the sun vitamin – simply because we do not get into the sun often enough – how many people do you know who leave home in the early hours of the morning and then are stuck in an office block all day, leaving only when it is starting to get dark?

Fortunately, Vitamin D deficiency is a fairly easy fix. It is said that you can get all the vitamin D that you need simply by exposing yourself to sunlight for 15 minutes a day, preferably indirect sunlight when the sun is at its highest point.

For many of us, that is luxury we simply cannot afford so we will do the next best thing. One of the earlier steps was open your curtains or walk outside as soon after waking up as possible so that your body's circadian rhythms can adjust. Now we are going to extend that step by taking a walk around the garden or around your block.

Walking around the block is better and I will tell you why – you get to feel more a part of your community. Don't just power-walk past your neighbors, greet them with a friendly smile. Over time, you will begin to enjoy these real social interactions.

Make a point of getting into a set routine – maybe you can walk to the local store to get your morning paper or go to your coffee shop to get a cup of coffee. Take a little time to chat to the cashier, other clients in the queue or the store owner. This in itself can help to keep you more connected with your community and help you feel less alone.

It is a sad fact that despite all the technology we have at our disposal, or perhaps because of it, while we are in constant contact with people we have a lot less real interaction – we spend more time tweeting about life than actually living it.

If walking around the block is not an option for whatever reason, do not stress, it is also beneficial to walk around your garden – you can look at new plants growing or paying attention to all the little insects out there. This can be interesting and relaxing as well.

If you have pets, take them along for the walk with you. If you have small children, you can use this as a bit of quality time with them as well.

Starting off your day doing small things like this helps you to reconnect with the important people in your life and can be a great way to help you stay grounded overall.

ACTION PLAN

1. Find yourself a comfortable pair of shoes to walk in.

2. Identify a route that will allow you to encounter your neighbors, rather than just speeding past them.

3. Alternatively, just get out into your garden. Buy yourself a pretty plant that you will look after as part of this project. You now have something to check on every day.

EXTRA Morning Habit #11

Have A Power Shower Every Morning

In Ayurvedic medicine, cleanliness is considered very important. Practitioners will often bathe or shower two or three times a day for health reasons. In ancient Rome, bathing was considered an extremely important part of the day – though not simply as a means to clean the skin. In fact, the Romans would generally rub oil onto the skin and then scrape the oil and debris off the body with a strigil. A function that could easily be accomplished in the privacy of their own homes.

However, as I mentioned before, the trip to the baths was about more than just getting clean – they made extensive use of hydrotherapy and saw bathing as a social routine.

In Japan today, bathing is also not simply a means to get clean – in fact, you will usually just wash up in the shower and then climb into the bath to relax.

Whilst we certainly do not have the time to spend hours at the local bathhouse as the Romans would have, or to soak in the tub in the morning before work, we can also make use of some of the benefits of hydrotherapy as well.

Showering in the morning is a great way to round off your workout and get your ready for the day ahead.

Making your morning shower a complete body boost by dry brushing your skin to start off with. All you need is a soft, natural-bristled brush to help you with this. Start at your feet and firmly stroke the brush up towards the heart. Carry on until your body is done but do not use the brush on your face.

This will further stimulate lymph flow in your body and will help to speed lactic acid away from your muscles at the same time – this means that you should feel less stiff and sore after exercising.

At the end of your shower, boost your circulation by alternating hot and cold water in short bursts, ending with a burst of cold water. This may be a little unpleasant at first but it is a fantastic way to rev up the circulation and the metabolism.

When you get out of the shower, dry yourself briskly with the towel – the friction created in this manner will help to remove any leftover toxins and will, once again, give your lymphatic system a boost.

Aromatherapy in The Shower

Add in some aromatherapy to really boost the effectiveness of your shower as a whole. This is easily done by dropping a few drops of the oils hat you want to use on a wash cloth and placing it on the floor of the shower when you climb in. the heat of the water will help the oils to evaporate and you get the scent and benefits of the aromatherapy oils without needing to apply them directly to the skin.

You can choose oils that help to boost your energy or, if you are feeling a little under the weather, you can use oils to help you heal. As a general guide, the citrus oils are very invigorating, as are oils like Rosemary and Peppermint.

Here is a list of oils that you might want to consider using:

Lavender

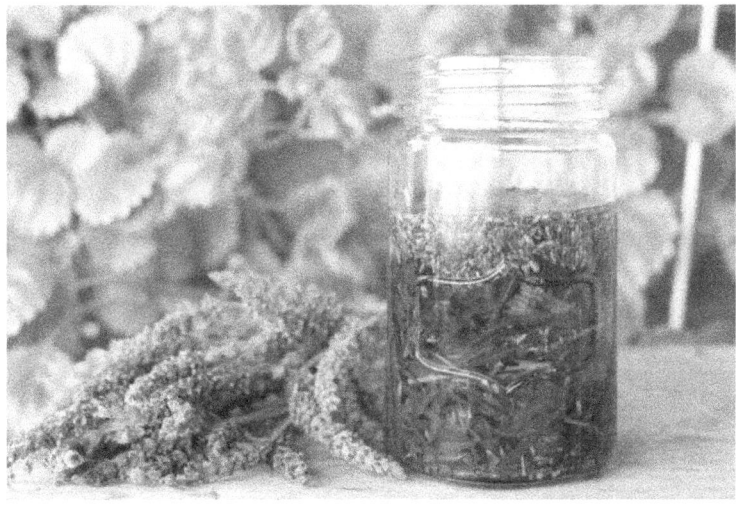

Okay, I am not keen on the smell but I do admit that it is quite a useful one to have around. A few drops in the shower on a warm wash cloth will help to calm the mind and soothe headaches. It also has an anti-bacterial and anti-viral action, perfect if you have a touch of flu.

Keeping the oil at home is good for other uses as well. It is great to apply to a small scratch or cut, it helps soothe an insect bite and I have gotten rid of a lot of rashes by using Lavender oil. What I do like is that you can apply it neat.

Massage in a drop or two of the oil into each temple and into the back of the neck to get rid of a tension headache or when you have slept in a funny position.

If you do love the scent, that is great. Apply it to tight muscles, let someone who has just had a shock sniff it. Spritz it on your pillows at night to encourage a deep, restful sleep.

Although classified as a floral scent, it is herbier in nature and so suitable for both men and women to use.

Tea Tree

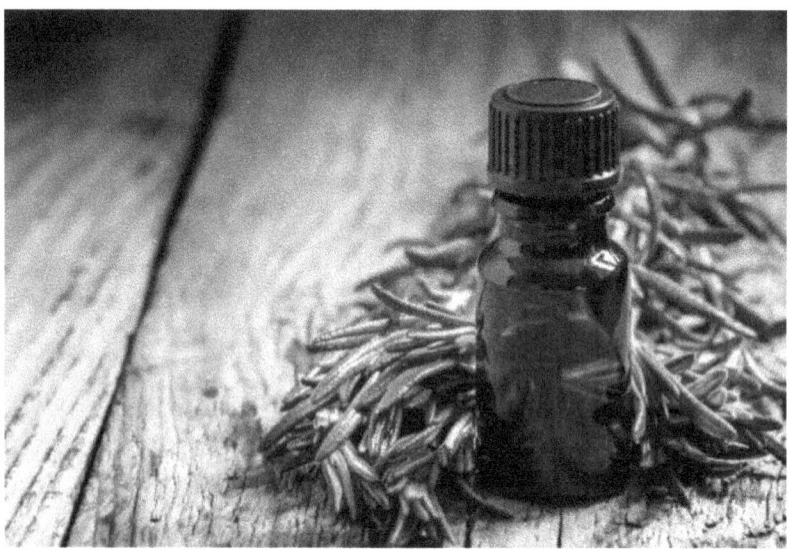

I am not keen on the smell of tea tree oil but I do believe that it has a place in a home aromatherapy kit. Sprinkle it on the wash cloth if you need to clear out a respiratory tract infection – it is particularly good when blended with Eucalyptus oil at fighting off colds and flu.

In the home, it has a myriad of uses as well. If I cut myself, I throw on some tea tree oil and forget about it. When I am neglecting my nails, I tend to get painful hangnails and apply tea tree oil to help them heal faster.

When it comes to fighting just about any kind of bug or virus, tea tree in the diffuser will help to sanitize the air. Apply a little to the sinuses to help kill off germs in that area.

Tea tree can also be applied neat - great when you are in a hurry.

Chamomile

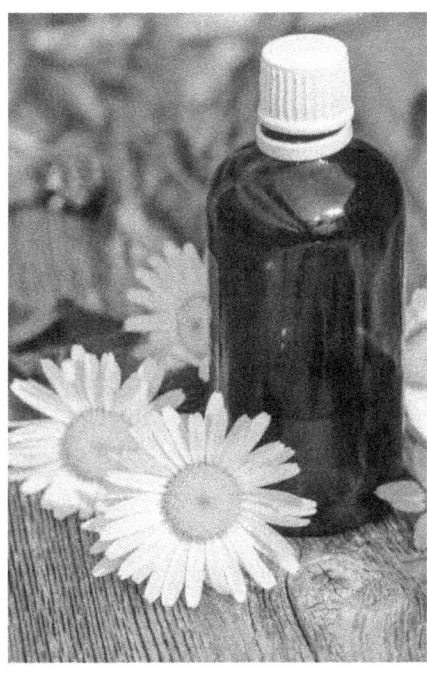

This oil does smell quite sweet so do see if you can find a tester before you buy some for your morning shower. On the wash cloth, it can help to calm and relax you – great after a restless night.

In the home, the uses of Chamomile are less extensive than when it comes to Lavender or Tea Tree oil but it does also have a place.

When it comes to pain relief, chamomile is my go to oil. It cannot be applied neat so do dilute it before using. I apply it to my cheek when I have toothache and it works amazingly well.

If I have a headache, I add a few drops of chamomile to some cool water and soak a wash cloth in it. Wring out the cloth and you have a perfect compress - if the headache is really bad, I might also add a drop or two of lavender.

I then make two compresses - one for the back of my neck and one to put over the eyes. Then it is off to a quiet room for a bit of a lie down - works wonders even with migraines.

Chamomile is also very soothing for the skin - rashes, especially allergic ones, respond well to it.

A bonus is that it also helps the skin feel soft. It is gentle enough to be used on the face, if diluted, and also by people who have sensitive skin.

If you have bad sunburn, or wind burn, or chapped lips, mix some chamomile, lavender and sandalwood together in an aqueous base.

Eucalyptus

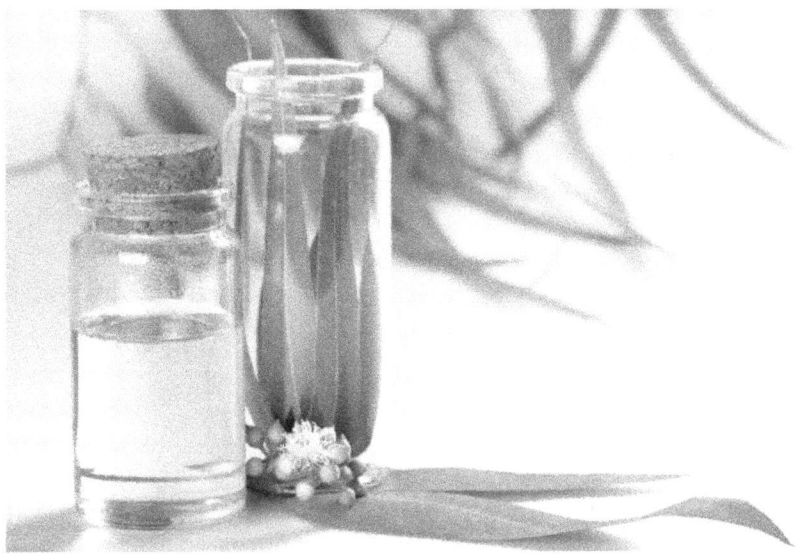

If you don't have this in your first aid kit, you are missing out. There really is no oil that is better for freshening up a sick room and helping to unblock a blocked nose. Mix some eucalyptus and tea tree oils and drop onto your wash cloth as a major weapon against all sorts of bugs.

In the home, this is another useful oil to keep - Mix some into an aqueous base and rub onto the back and chest to clear a tight chest. Rub the same mix into your feet, chest and back at night, just before bed when you have a cold or flu and you will feel a whole lot better in the morning.

Eucalyptus is also great for treating sore and tired muscles. Mix into an oil base and apply to sore muscles or put some drops in the bath or a foot bath.

Sandalwood

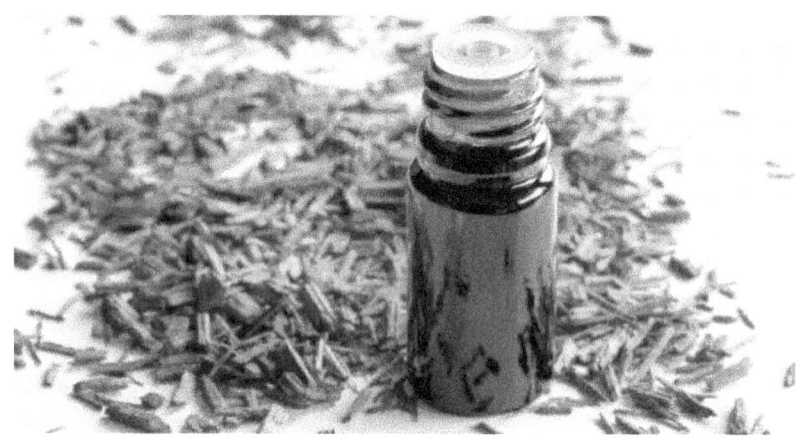

This is a very relaxing oil to use and it has a deep, exotic smell – perfect if you do not like the floral notes of the other oils. Sandalwood is a great healer when it comes to stress and tension and it is deeply relaxing. Add to the wash cloth and let the scent envelope you when you have had a rough night. Sandalwood blends really well with lavender and vetiver for complete relaxation.

I love sandalwood, I love the smell, I love the effect on my skin and I love how relaxing it is. This is a great oil to keep at home for uses other than the shower. If I am battling to sleep at night, a few drops on my pillow soon has me off to dreamland. It is also great blended with Neroli oil for when you are feeling stressed out.

For the skin, it is good for drier, mature skin that needs a bit of love and care. Mixed with Neroli oil and rose hip oil it makes a fantastic moisturizing treatment for the skin.

Neroli

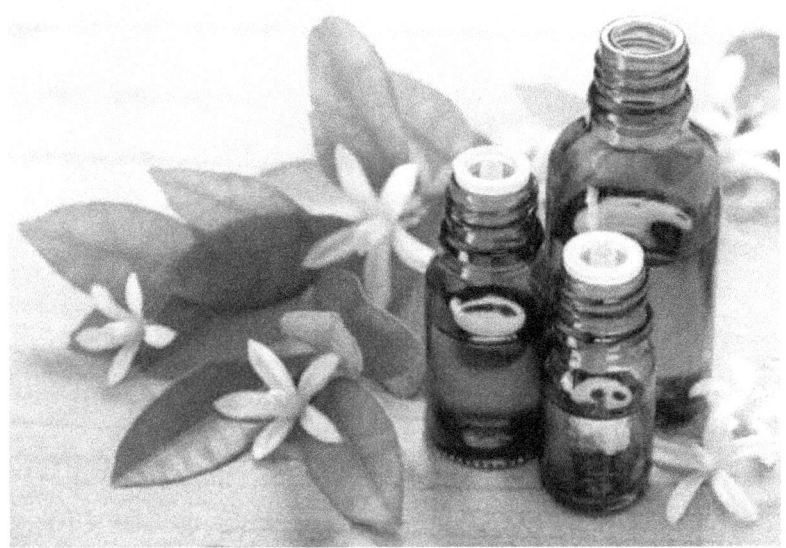

Again, one of my favorites - this oil can lift your spirits at any time and smells really good in blends.

It goes with most other oils so you will not often be without a partner for it.

Use when you are feeling really upset or anxious about the day ahead, or when you are feeling really depressed.

This is one of nature's anti-depressant oils and can help you to feel better in a hurry.

Benzoin

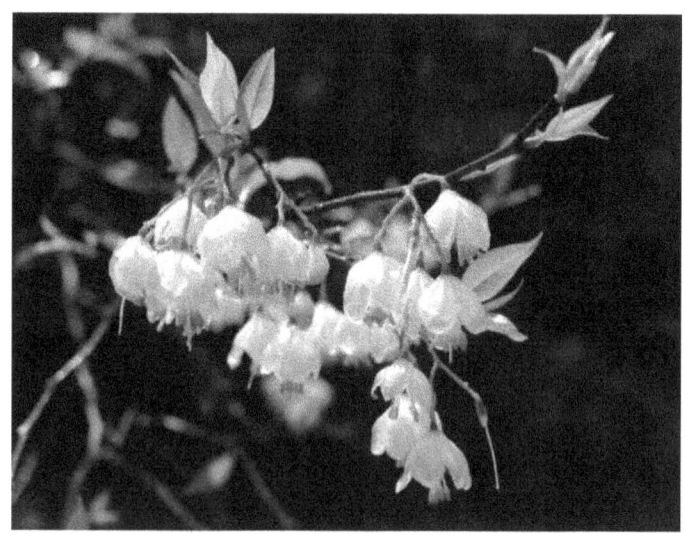

Benzoin may be a little harder to find but it can be worth looking for if you are depressed or if you have a stressful period coming up. Mix a couple of drops with some Jasmine oil on the wash cloth for a heady scent that helps to restore your feelings of optimism and ability to cope with stress.

Jasmine

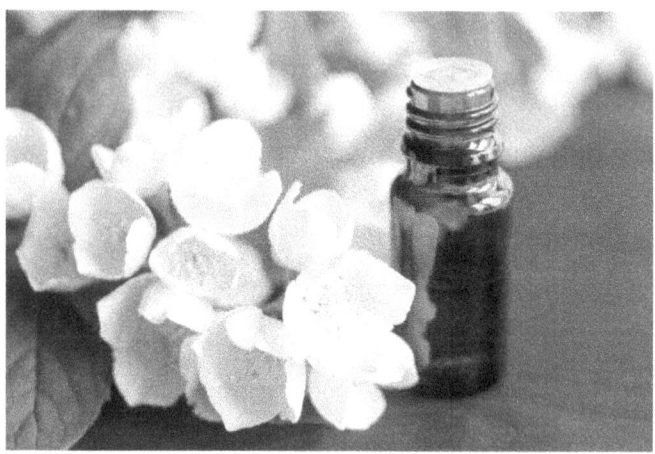

I do use a blend when it comes to Jasmine oil but it is one of the better brands. The extra expense is well worth it. That said, using Jasmine Absolute in the shower would be a complete waste because it is a very expensive oil. In this case, as long as you choose a reputable brand, you can get a Jasmine blend and use it with confidence.

Jasmine is another of those oils that mix with just about every other oil and it is wonderful to have in first aid kit. It helps create a feeling of happiness and will lift your spirits.

Use it sparingly as it can be a little overpowering.

Rose

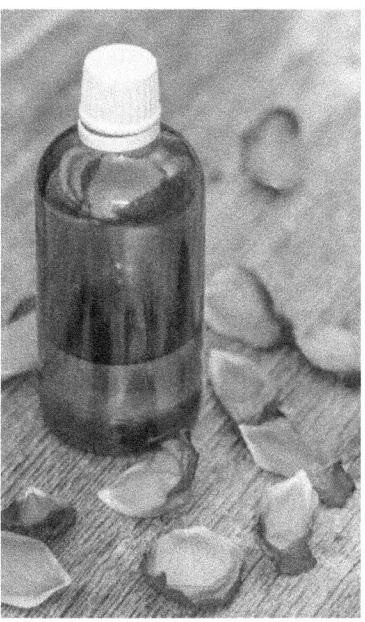

Again, I use a good quality blend because the absolute would just be too expensive. Like jasmine, it mixes with just about any other essential oil and lends a deep, exotic fragrance to the blend.

It is one of the best oils for dealing with stress and depression and to help restore a sense of optimism.

Ylang

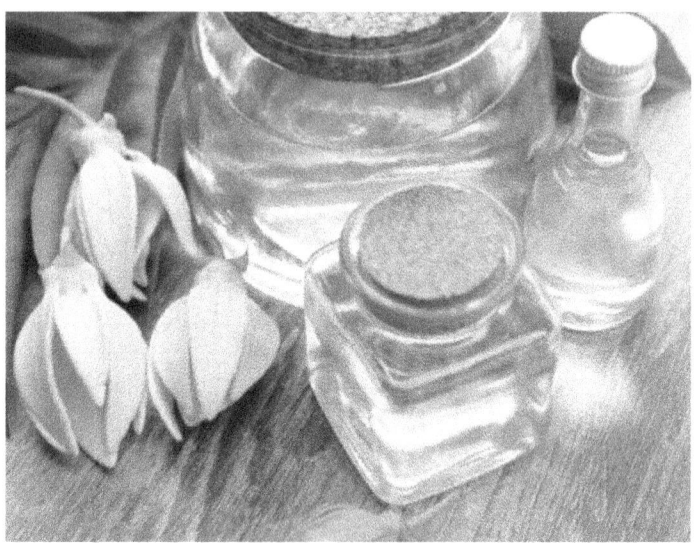

This oil can help you feel a little frisky so is a great oil to use in the shower if you and your significant other are planning to spend a lazy day in bed. It is also deeply relaxing so can be added when you are feeling under a lot of stress. You will either love it or you will hate it.

Ylang Ylang can be blended with Neroli and Sandalwood to give you a blend that will help you deal with whatever stress you are under. As it has quite a strong scent, add it last and only one drop at a time.

I do advise skipping the Ylang Ylang if you have a bit of a headache, as the strong smell can make your headache worse.

The oils that I have listed are only a smattering of what you will be able to find. These are ones that I use frequently but you do not have to buy all of them – choose a few scents that you like and then stick to those.

With aromatherapy, especially when we are applying it in the shower in this manner, it is especially important to find a scent that you actually enjoy. Otherwise the oil will be less effective overall.

ACTION PLAN

1. Look for a dry body brush.

2. Read up a little more on essential oils and find testers so that you can determine which scents appeal to you most.

3. Stock up on one or two essential oils – choose ones that you like and that will invigorate you.

4. Get yourself a wash cloth, if you do not have one already.

EXTRA Morning Habit #12

Find A Fitness App That Suits YOU

Earlier I spoke about looking at getting a fitness app like "Fat Secret" in order to keep track of your weight. Take it one step further by finding one that tracks weight, calorie intake and calories burnt through exercise.

Whether you download it onto your smartphone or you download it onto your laptop, the app will go a long way towards ensuring that you keep a firm track on what you eat, etc.

It can be quite easy to overestimate how many calories you use in a day and to become complacent about your weight, especially if you have been doing the morning habits for a while.

Every morning, weight yourself as normal and then also add in the calorie intake from breakfast and the calories burned as a result of exercise. You will then know exactly how many calories you have to play with for the rest of the day. This helps you to ensure that you stay on track with your weight loss goals – by both eating the right amount of calories and by doing enough in terms of exercise as well.

When you have found the perfect app to use, sync it up to their website. The disadvantage of only having the app on your phone is that there is only so much data that you have access to.

On my phone, for example, I can see my weight loss entries over the last few months. Online, I can see them since I started with the app a few years ago.

It is very encouraging to be able to see how far you have come – I remember looking at myself and thinking that I was "fat". What I found easy to forget at that time was that I had been a lot more overweight – having the computerized app, backed up offsite, means that it is accessible to you wherever you are. When you need a quick morale boost, check in and see how far you have come.

Most of the apps also allow you to connect with other users and have forums and "buddy" clubs – the buddy clubs are basically just there to allow you to connect with someone else that is in a similar situation to the one that you are in. The idea is that you will each encourage the other.

Being anonymous can also make it easier to talk about things that may otherwise embarrass you. Having the support of this online community may also help to keep you completely motivated.

There are also many of these apps that link up to exercise programs or that show you what exercises you should be doing via your smart phone. This can help to ensure that you do get your form in your morning workout right and can help you to learn how to take your exercising up to the next level.

You can, if you like, set up an excel spreadsheet to monitor all these stats yourself but it is a lot easier to use an app designed for the purpose. The apps make it easy to see what progress you have made and present it in visually appealing ways – you can do the same with excel but it will take a lot longer.

ACTION PLAN

1. Google "fitness apps" and look at a few different ones to see which you prefer. Look for one that allows you to track your weight, calories eaten and calories expended through exercise. Look at reviews of the apps to help narrow down the list.

2. When you have chosen the right app, look for it in the appropriate app store – many of these apps are available for free.

3. Download the app.

4. Register your account online and record your basic statistics.

I hope you have learned something from this book so far and would greatly appreciate it if you could leave an honest review on Amazon.com.

EXTRA Morning Habit #13

Mindful Eating

Ever had one of those mornings when you sit munching your breakfast while reading your paper or checking your emails? How many times have you reached down into the bowl only to find that you have finished your food without even really tasting it?

Food should be more than just sustenance and we need to spend more time enjoying the food that we do eat. You have, after all, spent a lot of time planning the perfect breakfast with the right balance of nutrients and healthy ingredients, does it not make sense to also spend some time enjoying it?

Mindful eating is a basic form of meditation where you concentrate only on the food that you are eating.

Really taste the food in your mouth, take time to notice the texture and chew each mouthful thoroughly.

Mindful eating is about making the food the primary focus during the course of your meal and this makes perfect sense – after all, what else should you be focusing on instead.

To help with the mindful eating, take a step back and start using proper dining etiquette again. Don't talk with your mouth full of food, put your utensils down between every bite and don't shovel your food down.

Yes, it is going to take you a bit longer to eat your food and it may be difficult not to multi-task at the same time but it is well worth the effort.

For starters, you will start to enjoy your food more and, as a result, feel less deprived. Focusing on your food will make you aware of nuances of flavor that you never noticed before, making eating a fun adventure.

Secondly, and perhaps more importantly, because you are taking longer to eat, you have a better chance of the brain's satiety response kicking in when it should instead of later when you have already eaten. It can take the brain up to 20 minutes to register that the stomach is full and so when you shovel down your food, you inevitably end up eating more than you should.

Finally, because you are eating more slowly, you are not gulping down as much air with your food and so will be less prone to bloating and gas. Digestion proceeds more smoothly than before and your stomach recovers more quickly after eating.

Make your breakfast a celebration – use your fine china and best cutlery. Pull out the nice table linen. You deserve to be treated well and so does your body.

ACTION PLAN

1. Starting today, start to chew your food properly when eating and really taste what it tastes like.

2. Brush up on proper dining etiquette and your table manners.

3. If you have no special crockery and cutlery to use, get a set especially for your breakfast meal – set the table, make breakfast a production.

EXTRA Morning Habit #14

Your Morning Pages

I first learned about the morning pages when reading "The Artist's Way" by Julia Cameron. I have to admit that when I first read of this exercise, I thought that at best it was silly and at worst a complete waste of time.

That said, the other advice in her book had been spot on – in fact, I do recommend that you read "The Artist's Way" if you do want to spark the creativity in your life. It is a useful book for you even if you are not an artist as it shows a different way of looking at things – you may even be surprised, perhaps you are the next Van Gogh. (That was my dream but, well, it hasn't really panned out like that – apparently, I have an artistic vision that is yet to be appreciate by the world at large.)

Let's get back on track – because the rest of her advice made sense, I decided to do the morning pages exercise as well. Now, it is actually a fairly simple exercise. You write two A4 pages of text without censoring it, without worrying about spelling, grammar, or even whether or not what you are writing makes sense.

The only rule is that you need to fill two pages and the work must be uncensored by the rational mind. This is a way to connect with the subconscious mind, a way to switch the rational brain off for a bit and to see what comes up.

The effects can be quite interesting. I will never forget my first line – "I have no idea what to write – this is so stupid. Should I write about my childhood?" and so on. What happened though is that I started to write about my childhood and I wrote about an incident at school that happened when I was quite young – the school had been showing the movie "Back to the Future" (okay, so you can work out how old I am) and I had bought tickets for my dad and me. He had promised he would be there but didn't turn up and I watched the movie alone.

Now, I am not telling that story to get you to feel sorry for me - what was interesting was that this had happened years ago and was not something that I really consciously remembered. It wasn't something that I had to go to therapy over and, if you had asked me if my dad had ever let me down, I would not even have remembered it.

My subconscious mind did remember though and it was obviously something that I needed to work through. Looking back now, I can see that this was one of the places in life where I started to have trust issues with people and now I am working through these.

And it is this that makes the morning pages so interesting for me – I never know what I am going to write about next and it is a really great way to connect with the subconscious ad bring issues that have been bothering me to the fore.

Of course, you cannot expect breakthroughs every single day. There are days when I fill a whole page with, "I don't know what to write about" and several derivations on this theme but the morning pages are something that have now been engrained into my daily routine.

It is also very interesting to read through the pages again at a later stage – I find it amazing how many patterns I have identified in this manner. For example, I figured out, through the morning pages, that a craving for a cupcake was generally always an indication that I was bored.

The morning pages can be tough to start off with – I am not going to lie to you, you will feel like a bit of a prat – but do persevere and they will become a really useful tool for you to work through issues.

I have also found that it is more useful to do the morning pages in the morning as this is when the mind is freshest and less full of clutter from a busy day. I have tried doing the pages at night before but found that then I tended to focus more on issues I had had with people during the day and generally found it more draining than helpful.

Always keep a pen with your file/ journal and always put it away in the same place every day so that there are no excuses to put off writing your daily pages.

It is better to keep these pages somewhere that no one else is liable to come across them. Knowing that no one else is going to read them can help you overcome the internal censor in your own mind. You can literally write down whatever you feel, even if it is something that you would never openly voice.

This can be a useful way of dealing with issues with other people without having everything blown out of proportion. You can work through the issues through this written medium rather than through direct confrontation and this can help you to sort through the issue more objectively – you might see that you have definitely over-reacted or perhaps identify an issue that you need to raise with the other party.

Either way, the morning pages can be a valuable insight into your soul.

A Dream Diary

Another tool that can be useful in contacting your subconscious mind is a dream diary. This is separate to the daily pages and can be explored at your leisure. In fact, if you have a rushed morning ahead, concentrate only on recording key areas of the dream overall. You can always come back to it later in the day.

You do, however, need to record the key areas of a dream as quickly after waking up as you can as these images can be fleeting.

Another way that you subconscious may choose to communicate with you is through your dreams while you are sleeping. Stephanie Meyer, author of the Twilight books, claims that the ideas for the books came to her in her dreams.

Think it sounds a little far-fetched? Well, actually it really is not. Think about it for a second - when you are sleeping, the conscious mind switches off completely - it is one of the few times that your subconscious is completely in control without the bullying influence of your rational mind.

While in this state, your subconscious works through whatever issues you have been mulling over, trying to make sense of them. Your dreams, therefore, can offer some interesting insights into your subconscious.

It can be very helpful to see what your mind has been thinking about.

Of course, that is easier said than done - dreams are fleeting and remembering them even 10 minutes after waking can be quite hard. Then the dreams themselves need to be interpreted - they are very seldom literal.

Remembering your dreams is something that you can work towards. Before you go to sleep tonight, say, "I will remember my dreams" about 15 times over. If you want you can also say what it is that you wish to dream about, especially if there is an issue that you want greater clarity on. Again here, clarity and focus is vital.

Put aside a pad of paper and pencil by the bed, and as soon as you wake up jot down bullet points about what you remember about the dream. You do not have to write every minute of every detailed account, merely write down some keywords or phrases that will help you to recall the dream later.

This is useful in two ways. For starters, it helps you to remember what you dreamt about and it helps to signal your mind that remembering dreams is important to you. Over time, you will find that it becomes easier to remember what you dreamt about.

When you have jotted down the key points, you can, if you like, write a more detailed account of the dream, or alternatively, discuss it with someone else. Both of these will help you to identify important aspects within the dreamscape.

When you have some time during the day, you can think the dream through in your mind again, even going so far as to ask questions or reacting in the way you would like to have during the actual dreams. These actions will all help you understand the meaning of your dreams.

There are a number of different dream interpretation books out there but I urge you to avoid these. While there are general themes in dreams, the symbolism in each person's dreams is different and so it requires a little more thought.

ACTION PLAN

1. Get yourself an exam pad and file or a journal to write in.

2. I find that it is most useful to glue a long length of ribbon to the inside of the journal/ file and to tie a pen onto that. This ensures that the pen and daily pages stay together. (Just make sure that the ribbon is long enough so that you can reach the whole page.

3. If you want to monitor your dreams as well, place a notebook and pen next to your bed so you can write down your key words as you wake up.

EXTRA Morning Habit #15

The Simple Way to Achieve Zen

Breathing is something that we do every day but also something that we tend to take for granted – after all, you do not have to consciously force yourself to breathe – your body does that automatically.

That is not to say that we all breathe as we should. Most of us have developed the bad habit of breathing too shallowly. Shallow breathing is fine, and actually useful if we are under a great deal of stress or need to get away from a predator – the breathing naturally becomes shallower so that we can get more air more quickly and this allows us to move faster.

The problem is that this is strictly meant to be a fight or flight response and not meant to be part of everyday living. Most of us, however, have become lazy with our breathing and deep belly breaths are no longer part of our daily routines. At best, we breathe with about a third of our lung capacity. (Okay, admit it, you just took a deep belly breath, didn't you? But when last did you force yourself to do that?)

The Benefits of Deep Breathing

Deep breathing involves filling your whole lungs with oxygen and then expelling all the air from the lungs again. The act of deep breathing signals to the body that it is okay to relax and your mind feels calmer. The benefits don't end there though.

The lungs are one of the primary organs when it comes to disposing of metabolic waste in our bodies. The carbon dioxide produced by metabolic processes is taken through to the lungs to be effectively scrubbed out of the blood.

From there, it needs to be breathed out. If you are constantly breathing too shallowly, your lungs are never completely clear of this waste product. Deep breathing is thus an important tool when it comes to detoxifying the body.

Of course, deep breathing also ensures that the body has ample supplies of new, fresh oxygen and the body is able to perform optimally because of this. You will fell healthier and more energetic overall if you practice deep breathing often.

How to Incorporate Deep Breathing

Now that you understand about why you should practice deep breathing techniques (though preferably not on the phone to your neighbor) you are probably eager to switch over to deep breathing all the time.

It is not quite as simple as that though – your body has had years and years to get into the habit of breathing shallowly and so it will be a tough habit to break. As a result, you are going to need to start practicing deep breathing techniques as often as possible.

Start with deep breathing every single morning until you get into the swing of things. Build up from there to practicing deep breathing exercises whenever you remember later in the day.

Eventually, you will become more accustomed to deep breathing and it will become more of a habit.

Deep Breathing Techniques

It sounds simple, doesn't it – breathe in and breathe out – even a child could do it. That said, there are a few techniques that can be practiced to make the breathing even more beneficial. I am going to cover some of these here and you can try them to see which you prefer.

At the end of these deep breathing techniques, it is common to feel a little light headed. This sensation will pass as you get more and more used to the deep breathing techniques.

Your need to physically feel the lungs filling with air, pushing out the diaphragm and abdomen. When you exhale, tighten your abdominal muscles to help you expel more air.

Breathing for Extra Energy

You can, even when breathing in deeply, tailor your breathing to be more energizing than relaxing. It is quite simple to do – the exhalation must always be shorter than the inhalation.

It makes sense to tailor your breathing towards building energy in the morning. Do this before you have breakfast – it is better when done on an empty stomach.

Start by sitting or standing up straight – good posture is important here – and breathe in deeply through your nose to a count of 5. Hold for a count of 5 and then release slowly through the mouth to a count of 4. Repeat 4 or 5 times.

Breathing to Focus the Mind

This is a little more difficult to get the hang of but it is a cleansing breath. It helps to clear out the cobwebs and helps to calm the mind.

Close off your right nostril with your finger and take a deep breath through the left nostril for a count of 5. Hold for a count of 4 and then remove your finger from your right nostril and close off the left nostril. Exhale through your right nostril.

Do this again, this time reversing the process – breath in through the right nostril and out through the left nostril. Repeat this exercise 5 times to start off with.

ACTION PLAN

1. When you lie down in your bed tonight, place your hand on your abdomen and breathe in as deeply as you can. Your hand should rise with your belly and if it does not, you are not breathing deeply enough. Breathe out deeply so that your belly becomes slightly concave.

2. Look up breathing exercises online to see how it is done.

Don't forget to share your thoughts on this book by leaving a review on Amazon.com. It takes just a few seconds.

EXTRA Morning Habit #16

Read Motivational Literature or Listen to It Daily

Do you know what one of the secrets of the super-wealthy is? They spend more time reading than they do watching TV. And what they read is important too – they read a lot of motivational literature. Now, whether you want to build your wealth or simply want to lose weight, the principle is the same – you need to read motivational literature. This helps give you the background you need for overcoming obstacles throughout the day.

If you are like most people, you do read some motivational literature already but I am willing to bet that you do not read enough of it or even that you read it every day and that is where the problem lies.

Read even one chapter of a motivational book and you will generally learn something – your enthusiasm levels go up and you become motivated to read even more. You may even end up reading the whole book very quickly.

That is awesome but what comes next? If you are like most people, myself included, you are all fired up for a while. Then day to day stresses start to take hold again and, before you know it, you have forgotten about what you read and are just trying to make it through another day.

It is hard to stay motivated when you are still trying to achieve your dream. It is tough to stay motivated when you are working at a job that you hate or are battling to pay your bills every month – I know, I was there once myself. Life simply becomes too hard and your mind gets cluttered with worries about paying the gas bill, getting the kids to soccer practice, etc.

And that is why we need motivation every single day. Even if it means getting up 20 minutes earlier every single day, you need to ensure that you read some motivational literature.

I have read all of Wayne Dwyer's books over and over again. I have read books by Louise Hay, Jack Canfield, etc. The list goes on and on. I also have several motivational audiobooks on CD and listen to those in the car when I am driving. In fact, when I used to commute every day to and from work, I would take that time to listen to my audiobooks and found that it was a lot easier not to feel stressed by work events as a result.

If you don't want to read the books, get the audiobooks and listen to them or get the DVDs and watch them. Each and every day! I don't care if you end up knowing the entire script line for line, watch them every day.

What begins to happen is that, after you have read a few of these books, you will start to notice that there are common truths present in all of them and that these threads are simple to pick up throughout.

This commonality reinforces the belief in your mind that these basic tenets are universal truths and you begin to apply them in your own daily life. Not only does reading the literature tell you what the truths are but it also tells you how to go about applying them to your own life and experience. Different teachers have different methods for getting you there but, at the end of the day, the basic destination is the same throughout.

And there is not a single excuse that I will accept for you not to be able to read/ listen to/ watch motivational materials on a daily basis. I will never forget having read in one of Tony Robbin's books that he was very broke at one stage but that he still found the money to buy motivational material. And look how that worked out for him!

The material is easy to find out there. You can buy Kindle books for less than the cost of a printed version at Amazon.com, or, if you are an Amazon Prime member, basically borrow the books to read for free. (Your limitation is that you are allowed 10 borrowed books at any time in your library.)

Do also look on Amazon regularly, Kindle books are often marked down to ridiculously small amounts or given away free in order to boost or renew interest in them.

If books are not your thing, head over to Audible and look at downloading some audiobooks. I find that these are especially great when I am driving – I now love long distance drives.

If you do not have the money to buy the books, go to your local library and see if you can find them there. They may be able to order them in for you.

Not sure where to start? Ask someone that you know is successful if they can suggest any motivational books for you to read – who knows, you might even find that they have a copy of the book that you want and would be prepared to lend it to you.

My favorite authors are:

- Wayne Dwyer
- Louise Hay
- Joe Vitale
- Rhonda Byrnes
- Jack Canfield

I find that Jack Canfield has a very nice style of writing – easy to read and get into and I would advise starting with his books to kick off.

That said, you can choose anyone you like, it does not matter who it is.

It does not even have to be in the "self-help" section of the library / store.

When I am in need of a boost, my favorite motivational movie is "Cool Runnings". It is a fictional movie but is based on true events – the first Jamaican bobsled team - and it is a really awesome movie. I have watched it over and over again and I love it every time.

On the other hand, I find Steve Covey's books to be extremely boring – whilst they have definitely got some useful information in them, they are just not for me.

Read books that motivate you – I can go on all day about what motivates me but, at the end of the day, it is you that matter – you need to find your own path. (And, if you haven't already, you do need to watch "Cool Runnings".)

The very last thing that I will say about motivational material is that you do need to be discerning in what you read – there is a lot of great material out there and there is also a lot of really bad advice.

Use your discretion to help determine what good advice is and what bad advice is – if it does not make sense to you, bin it. After all, if you think that the advice is bad, you are less likely to implement it anyway.

This helps you develop a winning mindset.

Developing Your Winning Mindset

We all face obstacles in life – what separates those who succeed from those who fail is the way they deal with those obstacles. Successful people will find a way to overcome the obstacles, no matter how long it takes.

Thomas Edison is said to have tried to solve the problem of the light bulb scores of times. When asked whether or not he should give up, his response was, "I have not failed. I've just found 10,000 ways that won't work." He did, in the end get it right – by doggedly trying over and over again.

People who do not succeed simply do not try hard enough to overcome the obstacle - they simply give up too soon. In many cases, they actually blame the obstacle for their lack of success. Have you ever said, "If I had more money I could've...."; "If I had a better job I would've". These are all examples of you shifting the blame.

Henry Ford Put It Better Than I Ever Could

"Whether you think you can, or you think you can't - you're right."

One theme that you will find coming up over and over again in motivational literature is the theme that you are in control of your own circumstances and it is important to remind yourself of that daily.

This can be a scary concept at first – you have no one to blame but yourself but in the end, it is empowering as well - No matter what circumstances you currently face, you will be able to succeed as long as you have a winning mindset.

Over and over we see proof of that. Look as Sir Richard Branson, for example. He came from a poor background, was really bad at English in school and left school early.

In spite of this, he still ran a successful newspaper. He built up a multi-million-dollar fortune and lost everything. He even spent time in jail. Imagine having nothing, getting it all and then losing it again. You would think that would be enough to crush anyone, wouldn't you? Well, clearly not – Sir Richard Branson has once again become one of the super-rich.

What sets him apart from others? If one thing does not work, he looks for something else – he believes that there always is a way to turn things around when they are not working for you.

And that is where motivational literature becomes extremely important – it not only relates the stories of others that faced tough circumstances and did well but also how they developed a winning mindset and how they never gave up.

It is kind of like the saying, "Winners never quit and quitters never win."

When I was younger, I made some very bad financial decisions and was dead broke. I had to move back home with my family. I admit to feeling very sorry for myself until one day it just suddenly occurred to me that though I had failed, I had done so in a spectacular manner. I thought to myself if someone like Richard Branson could lose millions and then come back from that, why should I be any different?

The minute I made the firm decision to stop feeling sorry for myself and to look for another way out of this situation, I started noticing more and more opportunities opening up for me.

I ended up recovering from the loss and learning to live a simple life – it was the best life lesson that I have ever learned.

That said though, it was not always that easy and there were times when all I wanted to do was to throw in the towel. Fortunately, I kept on reading my books every single day – even on those days when I did not want to crawl out of bed.

I cannot emphasize this habit enough – you need to motivate yourself to succeed every day – reading a self-help book once in a while will not cut it but when you incorporate making motivational literature a part of your daily life every day, you begin to let your brain know how important this is to you and it stands up and takes notes.

You can succeed at weight loss, at incorporating all the habits in this book, making more money, whatever obstacles you see ahead of you at the moment. Thomas Edison also said, "When you have exhausted all possibilities, remember this - you haven't."

Stop a minute and start looking at the possibilities – have you really and truly tried everything? The mind is your most powerful tool when it comes to being successful but you have to set it on the right track.

Stop blaming your lack of success on your circumstances. You created everything in your life – from the arrogant boss (you put up with his treatment of you) to the constant lack of money.

Accept that and move on as the director of your own fate, rather than relying on external sources to direct your fate for you.

Become A Winner Instead of A Whiner

It can be difficult, at least initially, to move from victim to victor mentality, especially if you have been in the former mode for a long time.

The first step is to visualize your life as you want it to be – to see, in your mind's eye, the success that you will one day achieve. Spend 10 minutes every morning visualizing winning behavior.

The next step is analyze your day to day behavior – are the actions that you are taking those of a victim or a victor? Let's say, for example, your boss berates you for little reason again – before, it would have ruined your day and you would no doubt have mulled it over in your mind over and over again.

How would a victor act? A victor, on the other hand would either tell their boss that they are not acting appropriately or, if that is not possible, ignore the hurtful behavior altogether. A victor would understand that their boss's behavior is the boss's business. A victor understands that they control how they react to the behavior.

The final step is to work on believing that you can be successful. If you cannot believe that you can actually succeed, you will NEVER be a success.

If your confidence is a little shaky, start out by setting small, achievable goals, goals that you can achieve in the next two to three months, with only a little bit of effort. The aim of this exercise is to build your confidence so the exercises should take you a little out of your comfort zone without being too hard to accomplish quickly.

As you progress and start to achieve these goals, your confidence will build and you can try to achieve more difficult goals. By setting mini-goals instead of huge goals, you get a number of different mini-wins that help to boost your overall confidence levels and help you to believe that achieving the goals is possible.

When setting your mini-goals, consider your end goal and use the mini-goals to help move you toward your main life goals.

Perhaps, for example, your aim is to be a conservationist and you currently work as a clerk in a law firm. Consider what skills you will need to be able to follow your dream career. What small steps can you take now to get you that little bit closer to your dream job? Perhaps you may need to consider part-time study, perhaps you can volunteer at a wildlife shelter – aim to do something small, every single day to help you achieve your dream.

Go through your list of goals every morning to remind yourself of what they are.

Affirmations

Now, affirmations can easily be incorporated into most parts of the daily habits – you can repeat them to yourself while exercising, or when you go out for your daily walk.

The point is that you now need to replace the old limiting beliefs that you had with the new ones that are more in line with helping you to achieve your goals. Choose one or two new beliefs at most in a two-week cycle – more and you will risk overwhelming yourself – and write them out in the form of an affirmation.

Make it as simple and easy to remember as possible and then commit to repeating it for at least 5 minutes a day over four to eight weeks. An affirmation that is a few words long is better because it is much easier to remember than one that is sentences long.

Many people try affirmations and say that they failed but this is usually because they did not persevere long enough. Remember, it is your subconscious that you want to convince and it is going to take some time to overcome a lifetime of negative programming.

If you work at it though, you will be find that the new beliefs actually become part of your own hard-wiring brain and it will slowly supplant the old beliefs. Over time, these beliefs will become instinctual and you will reap the rewards.

It is kind of like when you learned to drive – at first it was hard – I know when I first learned how to drive a stick shift, my leg ached and I thought I would never figure out how to change gears. Now driving is second nature to me – I can get from point A to point B without putting much conscious thought into it at all

ACTION PLAN

1. Get a library card if you do not already have one – many libraries also now have online lending facilities that allow you to borrow and read books online.

2. Sign up for a book discount service like Ebub – you get a daily email that lets you know about special offers in the fields that you have denoted an interest in.

3. Sign up for Audible – you do get a free trial period where you are allowed to download books to see if you like the way the system works.

4. Look for motivational forums to join up with and see what books the members recommend that you read.

EXTRA Morning Habit #17

Your Morning Meditation

Meditation has numerous benefits – it helps to calm you, makes you more focused and enables you to deal with stress better. Overall, if you were to only adopt one habit in this book, meditation would be the one that you should choose.

Now clear your head of any silly notions of meditation being a completely mystic art and being the province of yogis and spiritual gurus. Whilst meditation is an art form in a way, it is something that everyone can do, regardless of whether they are deeply spiritual or not.

Meditation, very simply, is the act of stilling the mind and it gives your mind a brief respite from the action of the day. Necessary in this world with its overwhelming reliance on constant stimulation.

And meditation is not something that needs to take hours either. In fact, if you can manage even 15 minutes at a time, you are way ahead of the curve.

Meditation is harder than you might think – just try this experiment for a moment – sit in a comfortable position for 5 minutes, set a timer to be sure of the time spent, and clear your mind of every thought. Every single thought. How well did you do? My first session was disastrous. I hated it. I simply could not stop myself thinking for that length of time.

The good news is that you can train your mind to become quieter – with practice it becomes easier and easier to enter the meditative state and you are able to maintain the meditation for longer.

The really great news is that there are a number of techniques that you can employ to make your meditations successful overall so if one does not work for you, there are plenty of others that you can try.

For me, the breathing exercise laid out below is the easiest form of meditation for me to accomplish. I find that it saves time to combine the breath counting meditation detailed below with the deep breathing exercises that we spoke about earlier. For you, something different may work a lot better – it all depends on your own personal preferences so do not be afraid to experiment with this one at all.

And do not worry if you only manage 5 minutes at a time at first – even with just 5 minutes a day, you will see some benefits. Look on meditations as a marathon rather than a sprint – you build your stamina in small increments and pace yourself as you go along, rather than sprinting all out to the finish.

Here are some techniques that you can try.

Your First Meditation Exercise

Sit comfortably somewhere that you will not be disturbed – somewhere peaceful and quiet. Switch your mobile phone off completely. Make sure that you are wearing non-restrictive clothing and that you are sitting comfortably in whatever position you find comfortable. If you are worried that you might over-meditate, then set a timer for 15 minutes or so. Just ensure that it is not one of those ticking timers as this can end up distracting you as well.

Close your eyes and breathe in slowly to the count of four. Hold the breath for a count of 4 and then release slowly to the count of four. While doing this, concentrate only on your breathing. If your mind wanders, gently move your attention back to your breathing and concentrate on the count.

Clear Your Mind

Sit comfortably and close your eyes. Take few deep breaths and picture, in your mind's eye, a huge white screen that takes up your whole field of vision. (I like to imagine a movie screen – I find that works quite well.)

When all you can see in your mind's eye is this white screen, picture a small black dot appearing in the center. Picture the dot growing until it takes over the whole screen. When the whole screen is black, picture a white dot in the center of the screen and picture this growing until the whole screen is white again. Continue in this manner a few times, until you feel calmer and more relaxed.

A Meaningful Meditation

Find yourself a place to meditate, one where you will be undisturbed for at least 15 minutes. Switch off your phone and any other loud noises in the room. You can, if you like, play relaxing music to aid you in quieting the mind. It is best if it is a soft background noise and music that has no lyrics. Identify a phrase that has some meaning to you – this will be your mantra during the meditation. For example, "Love is key".

Sit comfortably in a relaxed posture but do ensure that your back is straight. If your body is tense, you are going to need to do the basic relaxation exercise detailed above.

Close your eyes and breathe in deeply through your nose, all the time repeating the phrase that you chose in your head. It is important, for this exercise to ensure that you only repeat the phrase in your head and not out loud. (There are meditations that involve chanting but this is not one of them.)

Hold the breath for a count of five, and then release slowly through the mouth, again repeating your chosen phrase silently to yourself. Repeat this a few times and then finish off by concentrating on your breathing overall. Then slowly bring yourself back into things by opening your eyes and getting up slowly. Give yourself a minute or two before you go back to your normal day.

It is important, in the beginning at least, to do a basic review of how things went. This doesn't need to be a major analysis, just a quick check to figure out if this method worked for you. Was it easy to concentrate on your phrase or did your mind wander quite a bit? Was it easy to remember your phrase or did you keep having to think what it was?

Do not be too upset if this first meditation did not work as you had hoped it would. This is something that you need to practice. This meditation will also not work for everyone, so do experiment with the others as well until you get the hang of things.

Some Basic Transcendental Meditation

Get comfortable in a place where you will be undisturbed. In this exercise, you will choose an object to concentrate on. You can, for example, concentrate on the flame of a candle or a specific spot on the wall. It is best to choose a fairly generic item that will not evoke too much of an emotional response. (You can, once you have the hang of things, progress to an object that is has more meaning to you.)

Relax and start to breathe in slowly through your nose and out through your mouth. Concentrate on the item that you have chosen. If thoughts come to mind, let them pass without judgement, always returning your focus to the object that you chose.

Maintain this for a few minutes and then gradually allow your focus to shift back to everyday life. Give yourself a few minutes to get back to full consciousness again and then evaluate the success of the exercise as a whole. Again, do not worry if it did not work out exactly as you hoped it would.

Guided Meditation

If you battle to get your mind to switch off – as I do – a guided meditation can be particularly helpful. All that it is really is a set of instructions. Your guide will lead you through the meditation step by step evoking images of calm and serenity.

This is most often accomplished by mentally walking you through a peaceful garden or place.

Guided meditations can be found quite easily online – there are many free ones that you can listen to in order to get the hang of it.

I do advise trying one of the free programs and seeing if the guided meditation works for you before buying a program. Also, if you are planning on buying a program, do try to listen to a sample of the narrator's voice before buying it.

I bought one CD, strangely enough, by Louise Hay and the sing-song voice that she used really got on my nerves on that one. I can still picture the tone now and it still makes me grimace.

A Walking Meditation

If you are too restless to sit and meditate, you can engage in a walking meditation. This is a type of meditation that is widely practiced and has been revered throughout the centuries. It is the concept behind this that led to the development of meditation labyrinths.

Basically, the labyrinth is set up as a path that must be followed, with a complex design. There is only one path to walk on but the labyrinth twists and turns so that the mind cannot figure out how to "beat" it.

As a result, the mind gives up trying to figure it out and you simply experience walking the path and being present in that moment. The Chartres Cathedral Labyrinth in France is one of the most famous examples of a meditation labyrinth.

You can look into setting up a smaller model in your backyard or you can simply walk backwards and forwards inside or outside your home – it really depends on what you prefer and are comfortable with.

Start off by walking as normal and counting your breathing as you go along. Once you have established the rhythm, you can start to alter your steps in line with your breathing.

You might, for example, inhale to the count of four and take four steps at the same time. You can then exhale to the count of four and take another four steps at the same time. The number of steps is not all that important, as long as you are consistent and keep to the same pace throughout.

Whilst also monitoring your breathing, you can also take note of the sensation of your feet hitting the ground and your legs moving. Do not look directly at the ground but rather look slightly ahead of you.

It may be difficult to concentrate on both your breathing and the sensation of your legs and feet moving and, if you are finding that, you can choose to concentrate on just one of these aspects until you become more practiced at walking meditations.

Whether you are concentrating on the movement itself or breathing or both, do not let your mind wander at all and always bring your attention back to the movement or breathing in the present.

ACTION PLAN

1. Take some time out to try each of the meditation exercises listed above and see what works for you.

2. Look online for some free guided meditations. Simply google, "Free guided meditations."

3. Consider where you might want to meditate. If, for example, you have a rushed day ahead, you might want to combine your walk outside with your meditation – concentrating your senses on the walk, much like you do with the mindful eating. Alternatively, walk to a spot in the garden and meditate in the sunlight.

BONUS Morning Habit #18

Your Morning Visualization and Gratitude Session

Writing down your goals is admirable and useful. I read once that a goal that has not been written down is nothing more than a wish and there is some truth in that.

Putting your goals down in black and white makes them seem more real somehow. Sticking them up where you will see and confront them on a daily basis is a really strong motivational tool and is one that has been used to great success all over the world.

By itself though, it is not enough. The human brain tends to be lazy and, over time, you will stop noticing the list of goals. You will stop consciously reading them and that is the reason that you not only need to write down what your goals are but that you also need to visualize yourself achieving those goals as well.

Visualizing the goals makes them even more real to your subconscious mind and eliminates doubt about what it is that you want. Let us say that you want to own your own home and that you write that down as one of your goals. It is an admirable goal but it is a very vague one and, as a result, whilst you may end up owning your own home, it may not actually be the home of your dreams.

If, on the other hand, you picture the home that you want in your mind, creating a clear picture of how many rooms you want, what amenities you want, etc. your subconscious has a lot more information to work with and, as we learned earlier, more information is always better when it comes to the subconscious.

Your subconscious mind, remember, works differently to the rational brain – if you can visualize this already being achieved, your mind will see it as a foregone conclusion rather than a "want" and will work at bringing that to you. Your subconscious will be more open to opportunities and will look for ways to help make that dream a reality for you.

A Vision Board

Humans are visual creatures but it is not always that easy to create an image in your mind. Some people find it simple to picture things in their mind's eye and can actually see a visual image. For others, this is harder and they are better able to imagine feelings rather than a very clear image. A vision board is a visual representation of the things that you wish to achieve and can be a potent aid when it comes to your visualization sessions.

Look for images that relate to what it is that you want to achieve. You can find actual images of what you want or rely more on symbolic images – the decision is yours. Perhaps a picture of your dream house or pictures of the destination you want to visit. Make a collage of these images and put it up where you will see it every day.

Decorate it with objects that might relate to the dream as well. (My goal a few years ago was to visit London so I made a board with images of London and glued on some fun souvenir pencils that I had received as a gift from a friend.) Make it colorful and fun – and don't make too much of putting things in their proper places. Let your creativity out for this project.

Now hang it where you can focus on it every single morning.

A Daily Visualization

You need to practice this visualization for at least 10 minutes a day. If you find it difficult at first, that is fine – persevere and you will get it right. The more you practice, the better the results will be.

Visualizing your ideal life every morning before setting foot out of the door will help to remind you of what you want to achieve and motivate you to achieve it. This is a habit that you must practice every morning without fail. Once a day in the morning is fine if you are really short on time but twice a day can really help you to get the message through to your subconscious mind.

You need to actually picture what it will be like when you achieve your goal. Picture yourself as the top sales person, millionaire, etc. Create a mental image of what that will look like and how it will feel.

What will you do? The more vivid and detailed the picture is, the better. How will you feel? How will it feel to be a success? How will you spend your time? Remember the more detail that you can go into here, the better the end result will be for you as a whole. You can choose a specific visualization – showing you in your home, etc. or you can make it up as you go along. Do whatever feels right.

In all cases where people triumph over adversity, there is one common thread – obstacles are viewed as challenges rather than insurmountable. In many instances, these obstacles were actually viewed as opportunities.

If you want to build a winning attitude, you need to start looking at the obstacles in your life in a whole new way.

Turning Obstacles into Opportunities Through Visualization

This is not going to be easy – it is much easier to sit and think that obstacles are insurmountable – and looking for the good in obstacles is going to require a mind shift for you.

It is probably going to require a little creative thinking but that will prove worthwhile in the end – after all, your current way of thinking has not really paid great dividends for you so far, it is time to try something new.

Let us say that you have a talent for making beaded bracelets, for example and that you could earn some money by selling them. Perhaps you would like to take the next step but have done nothing about it because you do not have access to your own car.

The rationalizations for not starting your own business to date could be that you have no car to carry stock in, you cannot get to the local craft fairs or stores that you could sell your products at, etc. You believe that not having a car is the obstacle to your success.

Let us look at things from another angle. You do not have a car but do you really, really need one? Can you open a store online? Can you climb on the bus with samples of your product and then approach different stores to get orders? (Parcels could be delivered via bus or mailed.) What about opening a store on eBay or creating your own website?

You may not have a car but you are not without options. In fact, you may actually be in a better position because you do not need to worry about a monthly car payment, fuel costs or maintenance costs for the vehicle. That means that the biggest obstacle in terms of your success has actually been you all along!

Obstacles might just be the universe's way of telling you that you are on the wrong track and that there is a better way to do something. If something does not work out as you had hoped, it is probably an indication that this was not the right path for you. You may even find, if you look back on the situation, that you did something, even subconsciously, to sabotage the project.

At the very least, every failure is a learning exercise and so never a complete waste of time. You may even find that because of that failure, you are led to an opportunity that you would never otherwise have dreamt of. If you can see the opportunity in every obstacle, you are already way ahead of the curve. Being a winner means being able to make the most out of every situation – even those that are really difficult.

Keep this mantra in mind, "There is an opportunity in every obstacle." Look out for what you can learn from the experience and you will find a way to benefit from it. to you as long as you create a really vivid picture.

The Next Step – Gratitude for What You Already Have

The next step is to actually be thankful for what you do already have and it is best to do this exercise just after your morning visualization. Most of us are so busy wanting more that we forget to stop and be grateful for what we have. This ends up adding to our discontent because we will never always have everything that we want – there is always something new around the next bend to crave.

Feeling gratitude for what you already have will have a dual purpose – first of all, it helps to fuel a prosperity consciousness and, secondly, it helps to signal to your subconscious that it is on the right track.

Look around at your home, your family, you job and find things to be grateful for. It is not that hard once you get started and you don't have to worry about looking for big things to be grateful for either.

Perhaps you are grateful that you have a roof over your head or perhaps it is something as small as the stranger that smiled at you in the checkout line.

Every day, you need to look for at least 5-10 things that you are grateful for. Get yourself a journal and write these things down. Aim for 5-10 different things every single morning.

Do this for at least 2-3 weeks. You will probably be amazed at how many blessings you have in your life already and this, in itself, can help you to feel more content.

Also, by acknowledging what you are grateful for, you are predisposing your subconscious mind to look out for even more to give to you. The more grateful you are for what you have, the more content you will become and, over time, the less you will need to be content overall.

Conversely, when you are truly grateful for what you already have, and no longer feel the need to get more to be content, you will start to find that you receive even more to be grateful for – the universe is a very generous place and, if you demonstrate that you appreciate what has already been done for you, you open the way to receiving even more.

It is important not to simply stop at the list though – when someone does something for you, be sure to show them that you appreciate what they have done. This makes them feel good and more disposed to help you again in future but it also leaves you feeling good as well.

Don't be a schmuck when it comes to things that you have been blessed with. You have no doubt heard of the Law of attraction and it works with gratitude as well – if you are grateful for what you receive, you will receive more. If not, the supply may be cut off.

It also pays to share your good fortune with others and to have a generous spirit. If you cannot donate money or goods, can you perhaps donate some time?

Being of service to our fellow man is something that many people look down on but there really is nothing that is quite as rewarding as helping someone else out. It pays to remember the saying, "There but for the grace of God go I."

Sadly, I have found that it is often those who have the least to be grateful for that are more willing to be of assistance – simply because they understand a bit better about what it is to be in need.

It pays to always remember that a generous spirit is rewarded. If you are holding on too tightly to what you have, you cannot open your hands to receive more, can you?

ACTION PLAN

1. Start collecting images for your vision board and get a piece of card or sturdy paper to cover with it. An A3-sized card/ paper is perfect.

2. Look for images that represent what you want to achieve. Look for phrases that motivate you and use them on your board.

3. Your board is a constant work in progress so do not be discouraged if it does not look exactly as you want it to. You can always swop and change things if you change your mind about what it is that you would like to have on the board as a whole.

4. Get yourself a gratitude journal to record those things that you are grateful for in.

Discover Scientifically-Proven "Shortcuts" & "Hacks" to Lose Weight FASTER (With Very Little Effort)

For this month only, you can get Linda's best-selling & most popular book absolutely free – *Weight Loss Secrets You NEED to Know*.

Get Your FREE Copy Here:
TopFitnessAdvice.com/Bonus

Discover scientifically-proven tips to help you lose weight faster and easier than ever before. With this book, readers were able to improve their weight loss results and fitness levels. So, it's highly recommended that you get this book, especially while it's free!

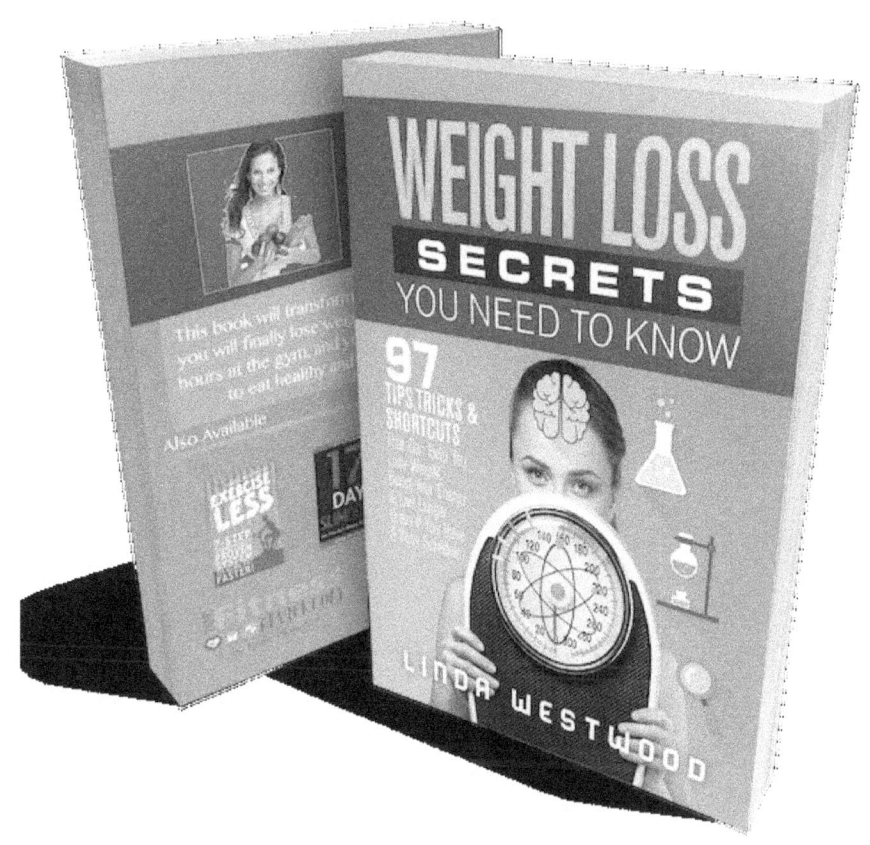

Get Your FREE Copy Here:

TopFitnessAdvice.com/Bonus

Final Words

I would like to thank you for purchasing my book and I hope I have been able to help you and educate you on something new.

If you have enjoyed this book and would like to share your positive thoughts, could you please take 30 seconds of your time to go back and give me a review on my Amazon book page.

I greatly appreciate seeing these reviews because it helps me share my hard work.

You can leave me a review on Amazon.com.

Again, thank you and I wish you all the best!

Enjoying this book?

Check out my other best sellers!

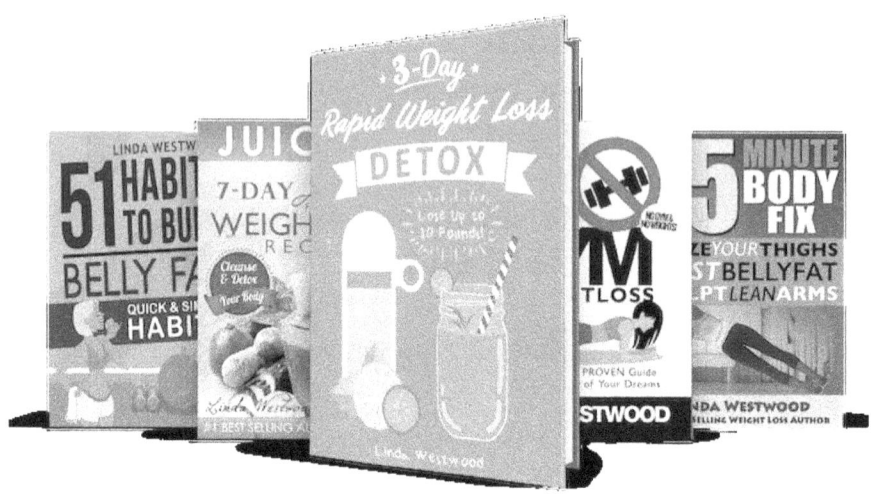

Get your next book on sale here:

TopFitnessAdvice.com/go/books

www.ingramcontent.com/pod-product-compliance
Lightning Source LLC
Chambersburg PA
CBHW020029040426
42333CB00039B/708